RETINOBLASTOMA – AN UPDATE ON CLINICAL, GENETIC COUNSELING, EPIDEMIOLOGY AND MOLECULAR TUMOR BIOLOGY

Edited by **Govindasamy Kumaramanickavel**

Retinoblastoma – An Update on Clinical, Genetic Counseling, Epidemiology and Molecular Tumor Biology
Edited by Govindasamy Kumaramanickavel

Published by InTech
Janeza Trdine 9, 51000 Rijeka, Croatia

Publishing Process Manager Vana Persen

Technical Editor Teodora Smiljanic

Cover Designer InTech Design Team

Additional hard copies can be obtained from orders@intechopen.com

Retinoblastoma – An Update on Clinical, Genetic Counseling, Epidemiology and Molecular Tumor Biology, Edited by Govindasamy Kumaramanickavel
p. cm.
ISBN 978-953-51-0435-3

For EU product safety concerns:
IN TECH d.o.o., Prolaz Marije Krucifikse Kozulić 3, 51000 Rijeka, Croatia,
info@intechopen.com or visit our website at intechopen.com.

Meet the editor

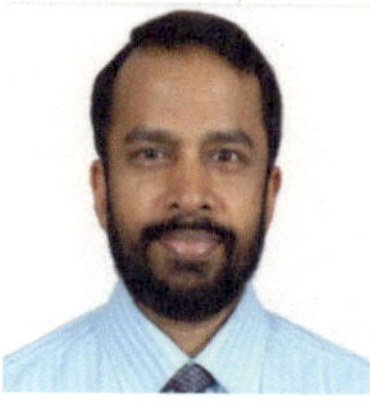

Professor G. Kumaramanickavel, MD, has worked extensively in ophthalmic genomics for more than two decades and has contributed significantly to the progress in the area of ocular genetics both nationally and internationally. He has worked on both single gene (retinoblastoma, corneal dystrophies, retinitis pigmentosa) and complex disorders (age-related macular degeneration, diabetic retinopathy, glaucoma), particularly in the area of gene mapping and was successful in identifying ocular genes. As a Fogarty Visiting Associate in 1997-98, he worked at the National Eye Institute, National Institute of Health, United States of America. Between 1992-96 he was a Research Fellow at the University of Otago, Dunedin, New Zealand. He is currently the Research Director at two eye hospitals in India – Narayana Nethralaya, Bangalore and Aditya Jyot Eye Hospital, Mumbai. He teaches at the Chinese University of Hong Kong. He has published more than 85 articles including Nature Genetics, Human Molecular Genetics, American Journal of Medical Genetics and Genomics .

Contents

Preface

Retinoblastoma is the first ever discovered tumor suppressor gene that opened a new avenue in the field of oncology leading to the identification of 35 tumor suppressor genes, till date in our genome. It is four decades since we know the two-hit hypotheses of Dr Alfred G Knudson and presently there is a huge amount of data available for us to completely comprehend the retinoblastoma gene and protein. However this reveals that there is more to learn and understand about its character and characteristics.

This book is an excellent compilation of both clinical and basic science information that meets the needs of a young clinician and a researcher at the same time. It also has abundant information on recent advances and cutting-edge knowledge in intracellular molecular cross-talking of retinoblastoma protein with various cellular viral-like proteins.

Looking into the details of this book, you will find that there is an excellent clinical description of the disease with adequate illustrations. The dreadful problem of second malignancies both ocular and non-ocular is dealt with elegantly. The ototoxic hearing loss in retinoblastoma patients provides greater insight into the disease, which would be a useful tool for practicing clinicians. For all levels of clinicians, whether entry, mid or senior, there is information on the genetic counseling and molecular diagnostics which are very useful. The epidemiology of retinoblastoma is a revelation for those both in clinics and research.

In understanding the molecular tumor biology of the disease, the role of RB protein in cell growth and tumor progression is extensively described. Interestingly a little known role of RB protein in the survival and differentiation of cerebellar neurons is discussed in great detail. The role of viral oncogenes and retinoblastoma family proteins is an exciting area that is teased out. The genetics of retinoblastoma is described quite elaborately as well.

Dr. Govindasamy Kumaramanickavel
Research Director, Narayana Nethralaya, Bangalore,
Advisor - Research, Academics and Management, Aditya Jyot Eye Hospital, Mumbai
India
Visiting Associate, Ophthalmic Genetics and Clinical Services Branch,
National Eye Institute, NIH
USA

Part 1

Clinical Sciences

1

Review of Clinical Presentations of Retinoblastoma

Onyekonwu Chijioke Godson
MBBS, FICS
Nigeria

1. Introduction

A retinoblastoma is a neuroblastoma. It is a rare eye tumor of childhood that arises in the retina and represents the most common intraocular malignancy of infancy and childhood **-1**. It may occur at any age-**2**, but most often it occurs in younger children, usually before the age of two years. Most affected children are diagnosed before the age of five years-**1**,**3**. Intraocular tumours may exhibit a variety of growth patterns and is commonly seen in advanced countries. Extraocular retinoblastoma is common in developing countries because of delay in diagnosis.-**4**,**5**.

In 60% of cases, the disease is unilateral (non hereditary) and the median age at diagnosis is two years. Retinoblastoma is bilateral (hereditary) in about 40% of cases with a median age at diagnosis of one year-**1**. Trilateral retinoblastoma is rare and refers to bilateral or unilateral retinoblastoma associated with an intracranial primitive neuroectodermal tumor in the pineal or suprasellar region-**6**. The median time interval from diagnosis of retinoblastoma to the development of a pineal region tumor was 24 months whereas the median time interval for the development of a suprasellar region tumor was 1 month-**6.** Untreated, retinoblastoma is fatal. In the developing countries, retinoblastoma presents with advanced disease with resultant 5 year survival of less than 50%-**7** whereas patients present with intraocular disease in the developed countries due to availability of resources for early detection and treatment. The survival rate in these nations has improved from approximately 30% in the 1930s to over 90% in the 1990s **-8,9.** In the middle income countries, the survival rate is about 70% **-10.** Retinoblastoma occurs equally in males and females and there is no predilection for any race or any particular eye-**11**.

2. What are the common symptoms of retinoblastoma

a. Leucocoria (white papillary reflex or cat's eye) is the most common accounting for about 60%- 80% of cases.-**1**,**4**,**5**. This is the most common type of presentation where there is high level of awareness such as in high income countries
b. Strabismus occurs in about 20% of cases-**1**,**4**
c. Orbital inflammation is seen in cases of tumour necrosis-**4**
d. Proptosis follows orbital invasion. Secondary microbial infections are often present. This is a common type of presentation in most developing nations-**12** due mainly to socioeconomic and cultural limitations resulting in delayed presentation **-10**

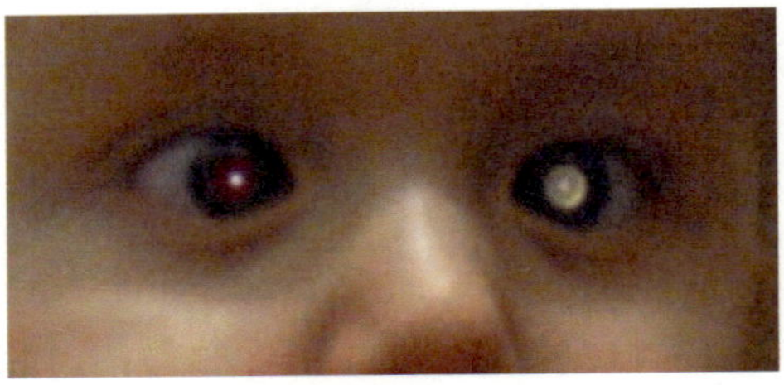

Fig. 1. Left leucocoria in a child with retinoblastoma. Courtesy. Wikipedia

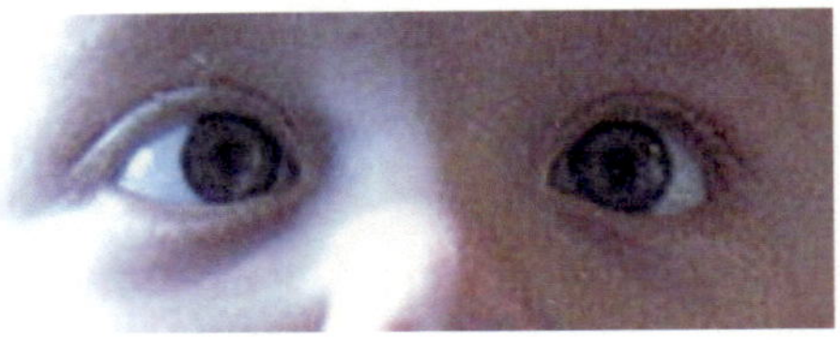

Fig. 2. Crossed eye in a child with retinoblastoma. Courtesy. Wikipedia

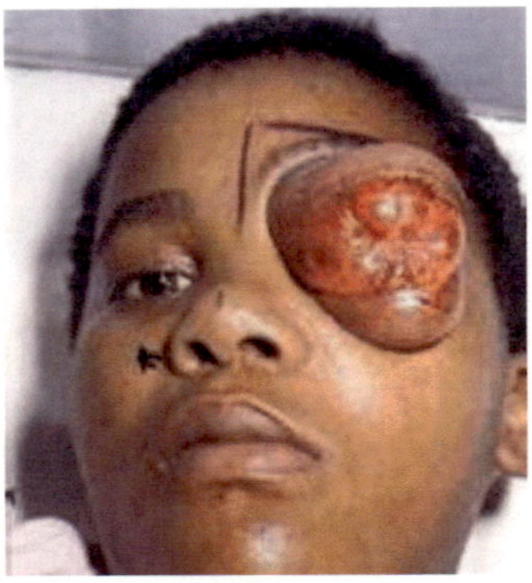

Fig. 3. Courtesy. www.arquivosdamorte.com

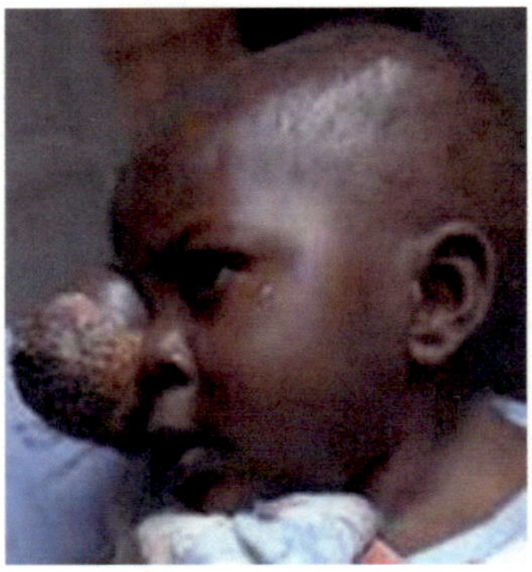

Fig. 4. Courtesy. projectmedishare.wordpress

Advanced extra ocular retinoblastoma in African and South American children above

e. Metastatic spread involves the brain/central nervous system, bones (especially skull bones and long bones), liver, spleen, Lymph nodes etc. This is worse in undeveloped economies due to late presentation and paucity of means of diagnosis -(**-1,4,5,12**)

f. Decrease in visual acuity-**12**

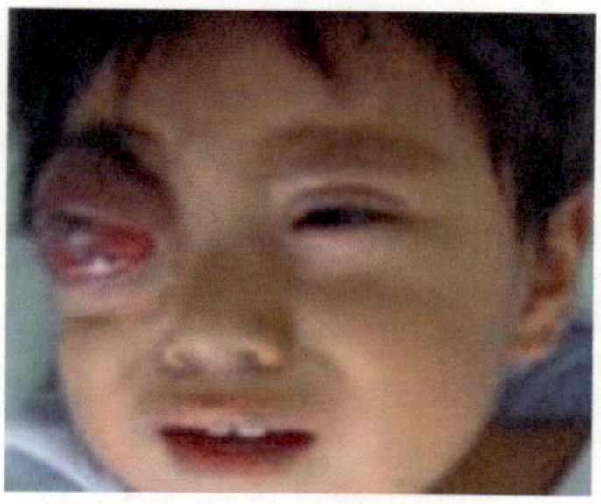

Fig. 5. Courtesy. inctr.ctisinc.com.

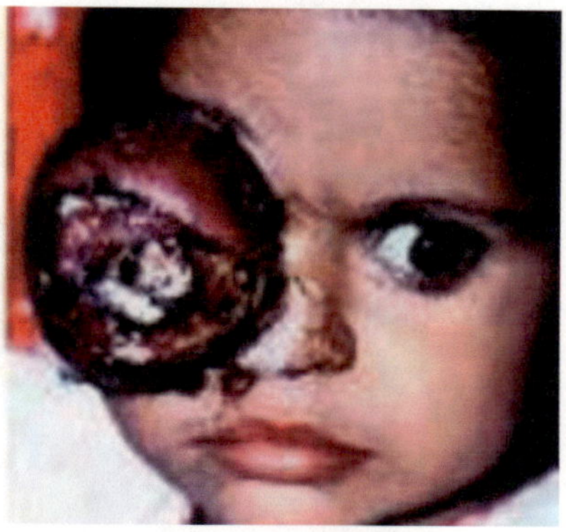

Fig. 6. Courtesy. www.jornallivre.com.br

3. What are the common signs of retinoblastoma

The clinical signs-**5,12** vary with the stage of the tumour at the time of presentation.

a. Early intraretinal tumour is a flat lesion which appears transparent or translucent. This type is commonly seen in high income countries where increase in awareness and early presentation are the norms
b. Endophytic tumour projects from retinal surface toward the vitreous as a friable mass, frequently associated with fine blood vessels on its surface-**4**. The tumour resembles cottage cheese if calcified. Vitreous seeding may be present

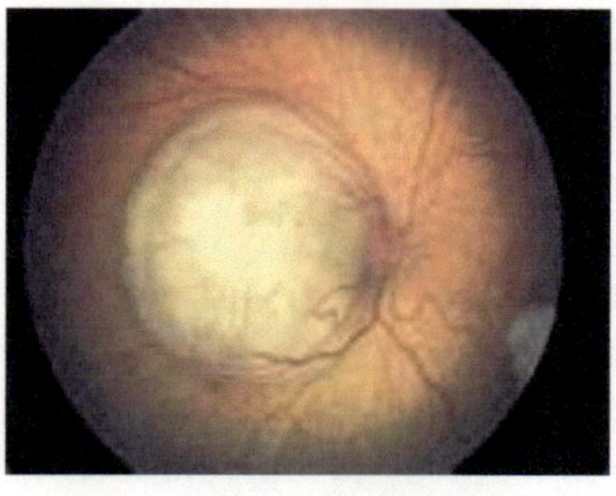

Fig. 7. Endophytic tumour. Courtesy. www.retinoblastomainfo.com

c. Exophytic tumour. This grows from the retina outward into the subretinal space with progressive retinal detachment. It may become a multilobulated mass with overlying retinal detachment. As the orbital structures are invaded, proptosis increases. Sometimes the grossly detached retina may be visible just behind the clear lens. Presence of vitreous hemorrhage may make the fundus hazy. Clinically, they may resemble coats disease

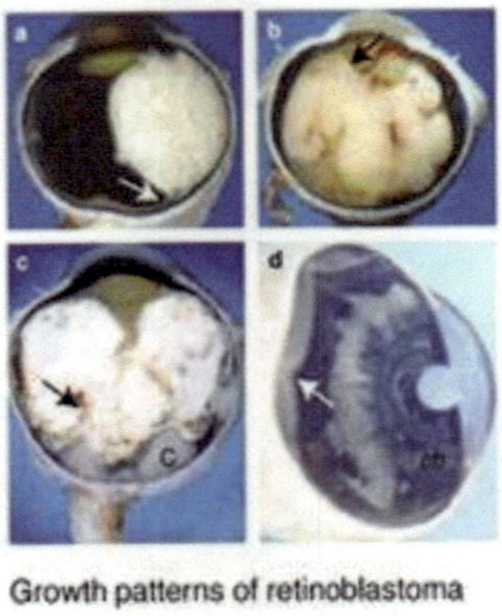

Fig. 8. Fundus pictures of Retinoblastoma. Courtesy. journals.cambridge.org

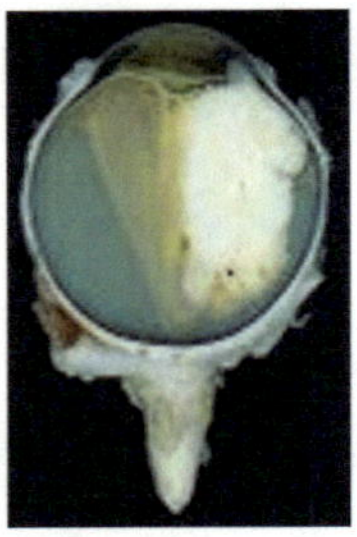

Fig. 9. Large exophytic retinoblastoma with calcification producing exudative retinal detachment. Courtesy. Wikimedia commons

d. Occasionally, a retinoblastoma can assume a diffuse infiltrating feature characterized by a relatively flat infiltration of the retina by tumour cells without an obvious mass. In such cases, diagnosis may be more difficult and this pattern can simulate uveitis or endophthalmitis

4. Less frequent signs of clinical presentations

a. Secondary glaucoma with or without buphthalmos-**4,13**. This is rare. Pain may be a feature
b. Anterior segment invasion-**4, 13.** Multifocal iris invasion may be associated with hyphema and iris neovascularization; painful red eye with pseudohypopyon due to tumour seeding into the anterior chamber. This is mostly unilateral involvement with no family history.-**4**
c. Associated conditions. 13q deletion syndrome has retinoblastoma, dysmorphic features, mental retardation which may be associated in some patients-**1**

5. Differential diagnosis of retinoblastoma

Some patients diagnosed initially with possible retinoblastoma prove, on referral to ocular oncologists and radiologists, to have pseudoretinoblastoma-**4,5,13** and not retinoblastoma The more frequently encountered being

Persistent hyperplastic primary vitreous
Coats disease
Ocular toxocariasis
Others include:
Preseptal or orbital cellulitis in extraocular spread
Cataract
Retinopathy of prematurity
Uveitis
Myelinated nerve fibre, optic nerve glioma, medulloepithelioma
Organizing vitreous hemorrhage
High myopia
High anisometropia
Retinal detachment

6. Classifications of retinoblastoma (Rb)

Several classifications of retinoblastoma have been developed to assist in prediction of globe salvage with preservation of useful vision where possible. There are two classifications for intraocular retinoblastoma currently in use.

1. Reese-Ellsworth classification. Originally used to predict visual prognosis of affected eyes and globe salvage after external beam radiotherapy. It is still useful to compare newer treatment modalities with older ones-**5**

Reese-Ellsworth classification of Retinoblastoma

Group i. Favorable

a. Solitary tumour less than 4 disc diameter in size at or behind the equator
b. Multiple tumours, all less than 4 disc diameters in size all at or behind the equator.

Group ii. Favorable

a. Solitary tumour, 4 to 10 disc diameters in size at or behind the equator
b. Multiple tumours , 4 to 10 disc diameters in size behind the equator

Group iii. Doubtful

a. Any lesion anterior to the equator
b. Solitary tumours larger than 10 disc diameters behind the equator

Group iv. Unfavorable

a. Multiple tumours, some larger than 10 disc diameters
b. Any lesion extending to the anterior ora serrata

Group v. Very Unfavorable

a. Massive seeding involving over half of retina
b. Vitreous seeding

2. ABC classification of retinoblstoma-**5**

To predict the preservation of the eye using all modern therapeutic methods

Group A. Small tumours <3mm (about 0.1 inch) confined to the retina
Group B. Larger tumours confined to the retina
Group C. Localized seeding of the vitreous or under the retina <6.00mm (0.2inch) from the original tumour
Group D. Widespread vitreous or sub retinal seeding which may have total retinal detachment
Group E. No visual potential, eye cannot recover

Others

3. Philadelphia Practical Grouping System of Retinoblastoma Based on Clinical Features.-**14**

To quantify retinoblastoma and its associated features without need to refer to complex qualification criteria. Proceeding from the lowest to the highest grouping is meant to imply worse ocular prognosis. This is a simpler and newer classification to Reese-Ellsworth.

Group	Abbreviations	Features	success*
1.	T	Tumour only#	100%
2.	T+SRF	Tumour + subretinal fluid	91%
3.	T + FS	Tumour +focal seeds SRS ≤ 3mm from tumor VS ≤ 3mm from tumor	59%
4.	T +DS	Tumour +diffuse seeds SRS >3mm from tumor VS > 3mm from tumor	12%
5.	High Risk	Tumor plus(any one) a. Neovascular glaucoma b. Opaque media from hemorrhage c. Invasion of post laminar optic nerve, choroid (<2mm), sclera, orbit or anterior chamber.	NA

*success after treatment with systemic chemotherapy with or without local consolidation is defined as avoidance of enucleation or need for external beam radiotherapy.
# Regardless of tumour number, size or location
DS=Diffuse seeds, FS=Focal seeds, SRF=Sub retinal fluid, SRS=Sub retinal seeds, T= Tumour, VS=Vitreous seeds, NA= Not applicable because these patients had primary enucleation.

4. International retinoblastoma classification

It is useful in guiding the selection of the most appropriate treatment methods and predicting chemo reduction success.-**15,16**

Group	Features
A	Small tumour ≤3mm
	Large tumour >3mm
B	Macular ≤3mm to foveola
	Juxtapappilary: ≤3mm to disc
	Subretinal fluid: ≤3mm from the margin
	Focal seeds
C	Subretinal seeds ≤3mm
	Vitreous seeds ≤3mm
	Both subretinal or vitreous seeds ≤3mm
	Diffuse seeds.
D	Subretinal seeds > 3mm
	Vitreous seeds: > 3mm
	Both subretinal and vitreous seeds > 3mm
E	Extensive retinoblastoma occupying more than 50% or
	Neovascular glaucoma or opaque media from hemorrhage to anterior chamber, vitreous or subretinal space

5. Classification encompassing entire spectrum of retinoblastoma disease stages-**17**.

This is an internationally proposed work to adopt a uniform staging system in which patients are classified according to the extent of the disease and the presence of overt extra ocular extension.

Stage 0. Confined to the retina. Eye treated conservatively.

Stage 1. Confined to the retina. Eye enucleated, resected histologically.

Stage 2. Confined to the globe. Eye enucleated, microscopic residual tumour.

Stage 3. Regional extra ocular spread. a. Overt orbital disease. b. preauricular or cervical lymph node extension

Stage 4. Distant metastasis. 1. Hematogenous metastasis: a. Single lesion. b. Multiple lesions. 2. Central nervous system (CNS) extension: a. prechiasmatic lesion. b. CNS mass. c. Leptomeningeal disease.

6. Extra-ocular retinoblastoma have 4 major types-**4**,**5**.

   a. Optic nerve involvement
   b. Orbital invasion
   c. CNS involvement
   d. Distance metastasis.

These are rare in developed countries such as the United States of America but unfortunately are still common in the developing nations due to delayed presentation and lack of access to proper health facility-**4.**

7. Racial differences in the time of presentations of retinoblastoma patients

An African series recorded a substantial delay before first presentation compared to what obtained in Europe-**11,18**. Essentially, many that delayed in African setting would have sought alternative treatments from spiritualists, traditional healers or quacks. Financial difficulties in funding treatment also caused delays-**18**. The series found a mean lag time value of 10 months in the study while the study done in London and Argentina showed lag time of 8 weeks-**19** and 6 months-**20** respectively. It was concluded that prolonged lag time is associated with higher risk of extra-ocular spread-**19**, **20**. Also, in the same study, disease staging at presentation was found to be more advanced in the African series and in India-**21** compared to what obtains in Europe and America. In Argentina, over 60% of the cases recorded had intraocular disease-**20** when compared with African series-**7** where majority presented with large extraocular, sometimes fungating disease(Figures 3). In developing countries, retinoblastoma is unfortunately accompanied by a high mortality rate due to a significantly delayed diagnosis made at advanced stages of the disease-**18,21,22**

8. Are there differences in presentation in children and adults?

Anterior segment invasion by diffuse retinoblastoma is seen in older children with average age of 6 years as compared to 18 months in typical cases-**4,5**. This is unilateral and nonhereditary. Retinoblastoma in adults is very rare. Age at presentation was from 20 years and above among the 23 recorded cases in literature.-**3** Clinical presentations were essentially different compared to those in children- **3**.

9. Laterality

Bilaterally affected children would carry one germinal mutation from conception and thereafter acquire the second mutation necessary for the expression of Rb. Unilaterally affected children would have to acquire two somatic mutations and this would explain why they would present at a later age than bilateral patients. The bilateral retinoblastoma patient present earlier in time than does unilateral retinoblastoma patients -**23**. Within early or advanced intraocular disease categories, the unilateral retinoblastoma patient will present later than does the bilateral. A series found that bilaterally affected children were diagnosed at an average age of 13months compared to the average of 24months for unilateral Rb patients-**23**. This average age for diagnosis of unilateral retinoblastoma is higher in developing nations-**18,21** because of late presentation.

Trilateral retinoblastoma patients manifest either as unilateral or bilateral diseases and are characterized by early onset and predisposition to developing secondary non-ocular, intracranial malignancies -**24**, **25**. Most cases of trilateral retinoblastoma, which occur in about 8% of heritable retinoblastoma-**25** are found in the midline pineal region, but they can also occur in the suprasellar and parasellar regions. These tumors usually occur several years after successful management of ocular retinoblastomas without evidence of direct extension or distant metastasis. -**26**. The nonocular tumors frequently present include intracranial primitive neuroectodermal tumors and sarcomas -**27**.

It is possible that many cases of pineoblastoma were previously misinterpreted as metastatic retinoblastoma to the brain. Unlike other second tumors, the pineoblastoma usually occurs during the first 5 years of life-**25** whereas second tumors often take many decades to develop, the incidence increasing with time, with a median age of17years (10- 32years)-**28**. The mean interval from the time of diagnosis of retinoblastoma to discovery of the intracranial tumor was 21.5 months-**29**. Unfortunately, pineoblastoma is usually fatal. Hence, patients with bilateral or familial retinoblastoma are advised to have screening for pineoblastoma using computed tomography or magnetic resonance imaging of the brain twice yearly for the first 5 years of life. In some cases the intracranial tumor preceded the diagnosis of retinoblastoma.-**25,30**.

Unilateral intraocular retinoblastoma associated with intracranial tumor was more likely to occur in patients with suprasellar region tumors than pineal region tumors ($P < 0.015$). The median survival after the diagnosis of an intracranial tumor was 6 months regardless of the location of the intracranial tumor. For patients who received no treatment for the intracranial tumor the median survival was 1 month whereas it was 8 months for those who received treatment. Children who were asymptomatic at the time of diagnosis of the intracranial tumor had a better overall survival than those who were symptomatic ($P = 0.002$).-**6**. Tumors of the suprasellar region present earlier than tumors of the pineal region after the diagnosis of intraocular tumors. The intracranial tumour represents ectopic foci of retinoblastoma rather than metastatic spread-**31**

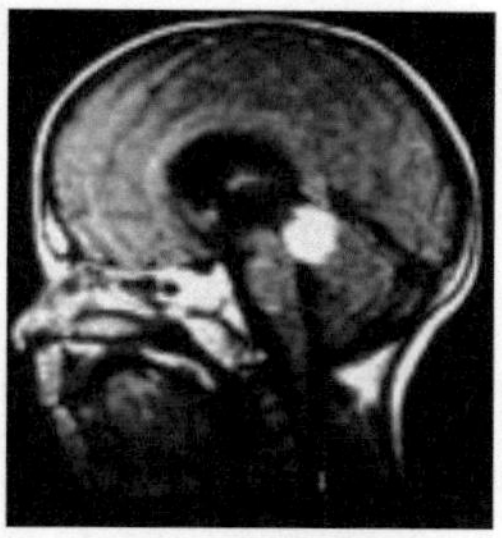

Fig. 10. Aspect of trilateral retinoblastoma on MRI. Courtesy. Wikimedia commons

10. A short mechanistic explanation for the clinical manifestations

Leucocoria is caused by massive replacement of vitreous by tumor and altered red pupillary reflex.

Strabismus is due to loss of central vision following retinal detachment, vitreous hemorrhage, glaucoma or optic nerve involvement singly or in combination.

Proptosis is as a result of tumour growth with displacement of normal tissues or seeding into the tissues and consequent enlargement of the tissues.

Orbital inflammation follows release of toxins from tissue necrosis.

Mucopurulent or fungating ocular mass results from mixed microbial infections due to neglect or mismanagement.

Convulsions and neurological deficits arise from spinal cord or brain metastasis.

Palor is due to anemia following bone marrow metastasis, oncogenic drug administration and radiotherapy

Easy brusability/ bleeding diasthesis are due to low platelet count following bone marrow involvement, oncogenic drug use or radiotherapy

Bone masses following metastasis may produce aches and discomfort

Headache results from raised intracranial pressure.

Blindness results from optic nerve involvement, retinal detachment, vitreous hemorrhage

11. Clinical diagnosis of retinoblastoma

Diagnosis is made from history, physical, histological and radiological examinations; blood chemistry, cerebrospinal fluid and marrow aspiration analysis.

1. Intraocular tumours
   a. Well dilated fundoscopy is mandatory to visualize tumours and classify the condition. It is done under general anesthesia
   b. Indirect ophthalmoscopy with scleral indentation after full dilatation of both eyes is a must. Tumours anterior to the equator are visualized **22**. This method determines:
      - The unilateral or bilateral nature of the lesions
      - The number of tumors
      - Their position in the retina (posterior pole and anterior retina)
      - The tumor size (diameter and thickness)
      - The subretinal fluid and tumor seeds
      - The vitreous seeding: localized or diffuse
      - The anatomical relations with the optic disc and macula.

All these parameters should be taken into account for grouping the retinoblastoma and for making therapeutic decisions - **22**.

   c. Ocular ultrasound detects size, location and extent of tumour**22**

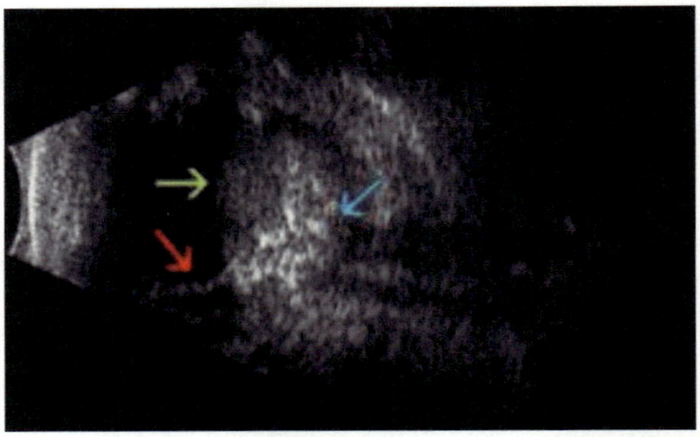

Fig. 11. Ocular ultrasound of large exophytic retinoblastoma. Courtesy. www.retinaatlas.com

   d. Cranial/ orbital computed tomography (CT) scan can detect intraocular calcifications and extent of the tumour-**22**.
   e. Magnetic resonance imaging (MRI) of the brain and orbits is the most sensitive means of evaluating for extraocular extension. It gives better delineation of the optic nerve and also the pineal area-**22,32**

f. Ultrasound biomicroscopy: provides adequate resolution of retinoblastoma anterior to the ora serrata in the ciliary region. Failure to detect anterior tumors early can compromise the chances of saving the eye and increase the risk of extraocular disease-**33**

2. Extraocular tumours
   a. Optic nerve involvement- MRI and histology

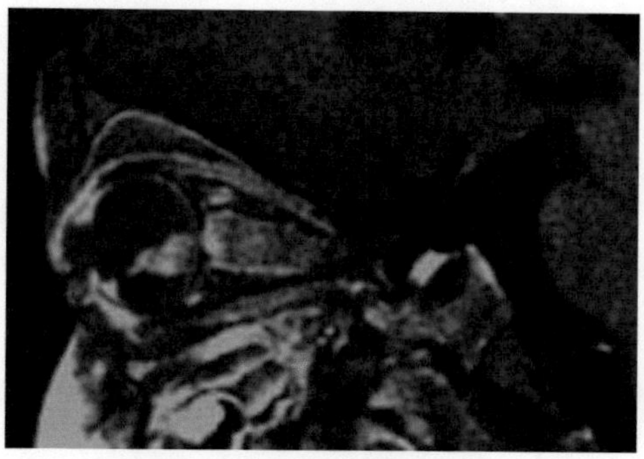

Fig. 12. MRI pattern of retinoblastoma with optic nerve involvement (sagittal enhanced T1-weighted sequence). Courtesy. Wikipedia

   b. Orbital invasion causing proptosis/lid swelling - orbital ultrasound and CT scan.
   c. Central nervous system (CNS) involvement causing brain and spinal cord lesions- MRI, CT scan and intracranial pressure.
   d. Metastatic disease-. Abdominal ultrasound detects pathology of the involved abdominal organs. During physical examination, Liver, spleen and bone masses and enlargements could be palpated.
      Skeletal survey
      Bone marrow assay
      Blood chemistry
      Cerebrospinal fluid analysis and cytology
   e. Non ocular tumours: MRI is the choice in detecting pinealoblastomas especially if a contrast material is added **22.**

12. Metastatic retinoblastoma

Significant differences were found in the occurrence of metastasis: in Low income countries (LICs), 32% (range, 12-45%); in lower Middle income countries (MICs), 12% (range, 3-31%) and in upper MICs, 9.5% (range, 3-24%; p = 0.04).-**34**

An average of 12 months elapsed between initial diagnosis of eye disease and the first signs and symptoms of metastasis-**35** Those at greatest risk for metastasis show features of retinoblastoma invasion beyond the lamina cribrosa in the optic nerve, in the choroid (>2 mm dimension), sclera, orbit, or anterior chamber-**35**. Optic nerve invasion was the commonest extraocular site of spread-**18**. Advanced extraocular retinoblastoma correlates with longer lag times from the onset of symptoms to the diagnosis-**20**. A study showed that at presentation, the mean patient age was 45 months (range, 13-86 months) and all patients with metastatic retinoblastoma had histopathologic or MRI evidence of unilateral extraocular disease characterized by optic nerve involvement, extrascleral extension, or both.-**36**

When retinoblastoma extends outside the eye, it is difficult to cure, even with sophisticated and intense treatments-**35,37**. The prognosis for survival is very poor in developing nations where these treatment modalities are scarce.

Of the 71 orbital recurrence cases followed up over a period of 3–208 months (mean 34.8 months) in a study, 60 patients developed metastatic disease (85%), and 53 of the 71 patients died from metastatic retinoblastoma (75%).-**38**. In developing countries, the diagnosis of retinoblastoma is frequently made at later stages of the disease when extraocular dissemination has already occurred; therefore, ocular and patient survival rates are lower in these countries than in developed countries-**34.** Metastatic spread is uncommon in developed countries because of early detection and proper therapy-**8**.

Presenting symptoms of metastasis -38,39

Eye: eye lid swelling, visible mass in the orbit, ill fitting prosthesis, Ocular deviation, bleeding socket.

Constitutional signs: lethargy, somnolence, fever, irritability, headache, anorexia, vomiting.

Bone: Pains in the back or limbs

Presenting signs of metastasis-38 ,39

Focal neurologic deficit/seizure/nystagmus

Mass on the bone, body, eye or orbit (proptosis)

Pallor, Easy bruisability eyelid ecchymosis, eyelid swelling involving contra lateral eye.

Nose bleed

Hepatosplenomegaly

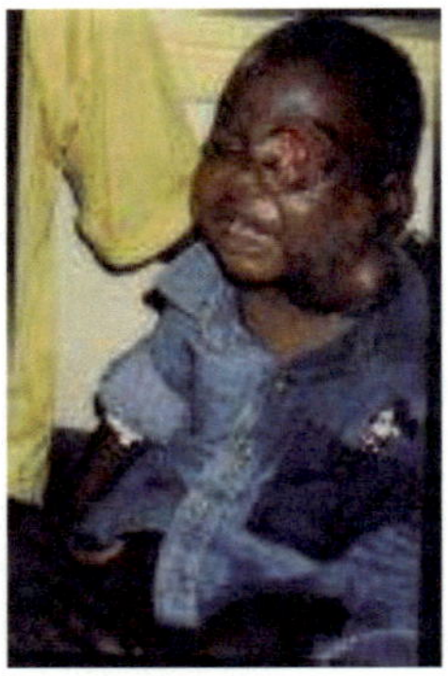

Fig. 13. Metastatic retinoblastoma in an African child. Courtesy. righthealth.com

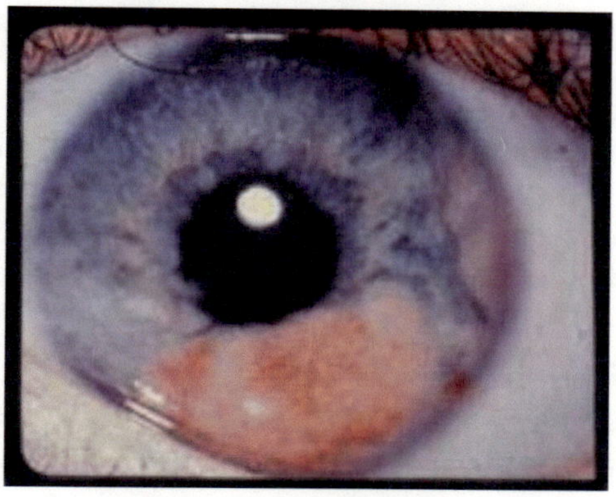

Fig. 14. Retinoblastoma with extension into choroid. Courtesy. www.thirdeyehealth.com

13. Useful tests to determine the extent of metastatic disease[40]

MRI of brain and orbit

Computed tomography scan of the brain and spine cord

Lumber puncture for CSF analysis

Electoencephalogram

Bone marrow aspiration

Bone scans

Automated blood chemistry analysis

Histopathology of enucleated/ exenterated eye, orbital biopsy, optic nerve and extrascleral extension.

14. Are some patients at particular risk?

1. Children with the heritable form of retinoblastoma are at high risk for developing subsequent malignancies, most commonly sarcomas. This risk is greater for those children with the heritable form of the disease who were exposed to ionizing radiation at age <1 year-**41.** The most frequent non ocular tumors encountered are osteogenic sarcomas of the skull and long bones, soft tissue sarcomas, cutaneous melanomas, brain tumors, and lung and breast cancer. Patients who survive a second tumor are at risk for a third, fourth and even fifth non ocular tumor-**42**. Subsequent malignant neoplasms are a major cause of premature death in survivors of hereditary retinoblastoma-**43**

2. Patients presenting with high-risk pathology features, such as microscopic tumor invasion of the postlaminar optic nerve (i.e. beyond the lamina cribrosa), choroid, or sclera, are at higher risk of extraocular retinoblastoma relapse. However, the relapse rate is different among the different groups. Such cases are more frequent in developing countries, occurring in more than 50% of children in some middle income countries compared to developed countries-**10**
3. Patients presenting with glaucoma and or buphthalmia have a significantly higher risk for the occurrence of pathology risk factors (PRF) including those resulting in microscopically residual disease. Major choroidal invasion and postlaminar optic nerve, scleral extension and possibly anterior segment invasion were considered PRFs-**44,45**

15. Recurrence of retinoblastoma tumours

a. Intraocular tumors may regrow after aggressive local and systemic therapy. Following chemoreduction and focal consolidation, tumor recurrence was found in 18% of tumors at 7 years and the most important factor predictive of recurrence was increasing tumor thickness-**14**.
b. The diagnosis of orbital tumor recurrence was made between 1 and 24 months after enucleation in a study (mean 6 months), with 69 of the 71 patients (97%) being diagnosed within the first 12 months-**38.**
c. Relapse. When analyzing patterns of failure in the 19 eyes that relapsed following external beam radiotherapy, a total of 28 failure sites were identified and consisted of progression to vitreous seeds in 7(25% of failure sites), recurrences from previously existing tumours in 10cases (36% of failure sites) and development of new tumours in previously uninvolved retina in 11 instances (39% of failure sites)-**40.**

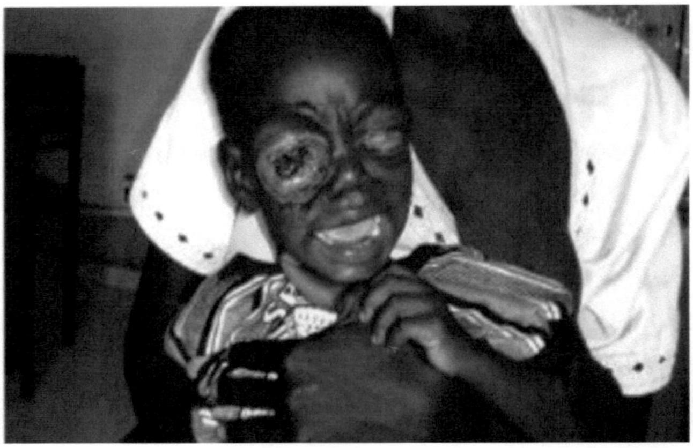

Fig. 15. Recurrent right retinoblastoma after enucleation in a 2 year old child with advanced bilateral retinoblastoma. Courtesy. Jacky Adura

16. Regression of retinoblastoma tumours

Retinoblastoma shows a variety of regression patterns.

a. Spontaneous regression of retinoblastoma is possible and may be asymptomatic resulting in the development of a benign retinocytoma or it can be associated with inflammation and ultimately phthisis bulbi-**5**
b. In evaluating retinoblastoma regression patterns following chemoreduction and adjuvant therapy, regression patterns included type 0 (no remnant), type 1 (calcified remnant), type 2 (noncalcified remnant), type 3 (partially calcified remnant), and type 4 (flat atrophic scar). The retinoblastoma assumes a smaller size with stable margins and frequently, some degree of calcification-**46.** Some tumors become completely calcified whereas others have minimal or no calcification. Following chemoreduction, most small retinoblastomas (3mm or less) result in a flat scar, intermediate tumors (3- 8mm) in a flat or partially calcified remnant and large tumors (8mm or more) in a more completely calcified remnant-**46**.

17. Retinoblastoma mortality – Prognosis

Mortality from retinoblastoma is increased in metastasis-**35**, trilateral cases -**25** and second malignant neoplasms-**47**, the last two are seen mostly in association with bilateral retinoblastoma-**48** and in sporadic unilateral cases that are hereditary-**49**

If left untreated, the mortality rate of retinoblastoma is about 99%. The major factor in mortality rates for patients with retinoblastoma is whether or not the tumor is confined to the eye. Extraocular spread increases mortality rates markedly. If there are tumor cells at the cut end of the optic nerve (with an enucleation), the mortality rate is much higher. Even if tumor is in the lamina cribrosa but the cut end of the optic nerve is free of tumor, mortality rates are elevated. However, when tumor is confined to the globe when enucleated, survival rates are greater than 92%-**48**

In evaluating long-term visual outcome following chemoreduction, the clinical factors that predicted visual acuity of 20/40 or better were a tumor margin at least 3 mm from the foveola and optic disc and an absence of subretinal fluid-**22,50**. Retaining visual function depends on the tumor size and location-**48**.

Over 95% of children with retinoblastoma in the United States and other medically developed nations survive their malignancy, whereas approximately 50% survive worldwide-**22**. This discrepancy is largely due to earlier detection in the United States and developed nations when the tumor is confined to the eye, whereas in underdeveloped regions, retinoblastoma is often detected after it has invaded the orbit or brain-**51**. The survival rate of patients with retinoblastoma is low in Nigerian, an underdeveloped nation, due to high mortality associated with late presentation and poor facility for detection and treatment-**52** unlike in developed countries. Again, in some African or Asian countries, the survival rate is virtually zero, because most patients do not complete therapy or are lost to follow-up-**53**. The mean interval from diagnosis of the ocular tumor to death was 46 months and from diagnosis of the intracranial tumor to death was 17 months-**29**

18. Late adverse effects of therapy for retinoblastoma[54,55]

1. Patients who received external beam irradiation are at risk for the development of secondary tumors within and outside the field of treatment. Radiation optic neuropathy and retinopathy can occur. Patients can experience ocular surface abnormalities, severe dry eye and cataracts. Radiation can also affect growing orbital bones, producing facial hypoplasia and contracted socket. Pituitary dysfunction may occur.
2. Chemotherapeutic agents are known to produce numerous potential side-effects. These include lowered immune status, increased incidence of secondary leukemia, infertility; auditory, cardiac, gonadal and renal dysfunction.
3. Cryotherapy can cause retinal thinning and retinal holes. This can be followed by retinal detachment, vitreous hemorrhages, tumor seeding and cataract.
4. Laser treatments can be associated with iris burns, vitreous hemorrhage, and tumor break with vitreous seeding.
5. Intra arterial chemotherapy: Risks associated with general anaesthesia, bleeding from arterial puncture, hematoma or arterial thrombus; drop in vision or total loss of vision in the affected eye, 3rd nerve palsy and sometimes risk of cerebrovascular accident
6. Psychological/Visual effects. The child may be blind from enucleation or from the disease itself. The child may present with low self esteem, limited social function and limited educational attainment.

   Another study showed that vitreoretinal complications occurred in 6.8% of patients undergoing therapy for retinoblastoma. These included retinal tears, rhegmatogenous and tractional retinal detachment, subretinal fibrosis, vitreous traction bands, preretinal fibrosis and pseudo-vitreous seeding. They were more often seen when systemic chemotherapy was combined with external beam radiation, cryotherapy and local chemotherapy-**56.**

19. Complication of retinoblastoma

Metastasis to the orbit, the optic nerve and then to the central nervous system. Other distant spread may involve the abdominal organs, bones and lymph nodes.

Loss of eye in enucleation

Blindness

Cosmetic deformity from enucleation, prosthesis and potential orbital hypoplasia secondary to external beam radiation therapy.

Second malignancy. This is mainly seen in patients with bilateral retinoblastoma who receive external beam radiation therapy-**55.**

Life threatening especially in advanced cases.

20. References

[1] Abramson DH, Schefler AC. Update on retinoblastoma. Retina. 2004; 24(6):828–848. doi: 10.1097/00006982-200412000-00002.

[2] Biswas J, Mani B, Shanmugan MP, Patwardhan D, Kumar KS, Badrinath SS. Retinoblastoma in adults: Report of three cases and review of literature. Surv Ophthalmol 2000; 44:409-14.

[3] Odashiro AN, Pereira PR, de Souza Filho JP, Cruess SR, Burnier MN Jr. Retinoblastoma in an adult: Case report and literature review. Can J Ophthalmol. 2005; 40:188–91. [PubMed]

[4] Jack J Kanski. Clinical ophthalmology. A systematic approach. Fourth edition. 1999. 337-339.Butterworth Heinemann. Oxford

[5] American academy of ophthalmology. Pediatric ophthalmology and strabismus. Section 6. Basic and clinical science course. 2008- 2009. 390- 399.

[6] Paulino AC. Trilateral retinoblastoma: Is the location of the intracranial tumour important? Cancer. 1999; 86:135-141.

[7] Bowman RJC, Mafwiri M, Luthert P, Luande J ,Wood M. Outcome of Retinoblastoma in East Africa. Pediatric Blood Cancer 2008; 50: 160- 162

[8] MacCarthy A, Draper GJ, Steliarova- Foucher E. Retinoblastoma incidence and survival in European children (1974- 1999). Report from Automated Childhood Cancer Information System Project. Eur J Cancer 2006 Sep; 42(13):2092- 102.

[9] Berman EL, Donaldson CE, GibLin M, Martin FJ. Outcomes in Retinoblastoma. 1974-2005. The children's Hospital ,Westmead. Clin Experiment Ophthalmol . 2007; jan-Feb. 35(1):5- 12.

[10] Chantada G L, Qaddoumi I, Canturk S, Khetan V, Ma Z, Kimani K, Yeniad B, Sultan I, Sitorus, RS, Tacyildiz N, Abramson DH. Strategies to manage retinoblastoma in developing countries. Pediatric Blood & Cancer 2011; 56: 341–348. doi: 10.1002/pbc.22843

[11] San SM, Lee SB, Au Eong KG and Chia KS. Incidence and Survival characteristics of Retinoblastoma in Singapore from 1968-1995. J Pediatr Ophthalmol Strabismus 2000; 37(2):87–93

[12] Akimbo WA et al. Presenting signs of retinoblastoma in Congolese patients. Bull Soc Berge Ophthalmolo 2002: 283:37- 41

[13] Balmer A, Munier F. Differential diagnosis of leukocoria and strabismus, first presenting signs of retinoblastoma. Clin Ophthalmol. 2007; 1(4): 431–439.

[14] Shields CL, Mashayekhi A, Demirci H, Meadows A, Shields JA. Practical Approach to management of Retinoblastoma. Arch Ophthalmol 2004;122: 729- 735

[15] Shields CL, Au AK, Czyz C et al. International Classification of Retinoblastoma predicts chemoreduction success. Presented at the International Society of Ocular Oncology; Sept 1- 5. 2005. Whistler, Canada and American Academy of Ophthalmology; Oct. 14- 16, 2005

[16] Saleh A. International classification of retinoblastoma. Saudi J Ophthalmol 2006; 20:3.161- 2

[17] Chantanda G, Doz F, Antonelli CBG, Grundy R, Dunkell I J, Gabrowski E et al. A proposal for international retinoblastoma staging system. Pediatric blood Cancer 2006; 47:801-805

[18] Essuman V, Ntim-Amponsah CT, Renner L, Akafor S, Edusei L. Presentation of retinoblastoma at a paediatric eye clinic in Ghana. Ghana med J 2010; 14(1): 10- 14

[19] Goddard AG, Kingston JE, Hungarford JE. Delay in diagnosis of Retinoblastoma. Risk factors and treatment outcome. Br J Ophthalmol 1999; 83: 1320- 1323.

[20] Chantanda G, Fandino A, Manzitti J. et al. Late diagnosis of Retinoblastoma in a developing country. Arch Dis Childhood 1999; 80: 171- 174.

[21] Sahu S, Banavali SD, Pai SK, Nair CN, Kurkure PA, Motwani SA, Advani SH. Retinoblastoma problems and perspectives from India. Pediatr Hematol Oncol. 1998; Nov – Dec. 15 (6): 501- 8

[22] Isabelle A, Livia L, Marion G, Hervé B, François D, Laurence D. Retinoblastom. Orphanet J Rare Dis. 2006; 1: 31. Published online 2006 August 25. doi: 10.1186/1750-1172-1-31

[23] Abramson DH, Frank CM, Susman M et al. Presenting signs of retinoblastoma. J Pediatr 1998; 132:505–508.[CrossRef][Medline]

[24] Abramson DH. Second nonocular cancers in retinoblastoma: a unified hypothesis- The Franceschetti Lecture. Ophthalmic Genetics.1999; 20:193 -204.

[25] Kivela T. Trilateral retinoblastoma: a meta-analysis of hereditary retinoblastoma associated with primary ectopic intracranial retinoblastoma. Journal of Clinical Oncology. 1999; 17:1829-1837.

[26] Cho EY, Suh YL, Shin HJ. Trilateral retinoblastoma: a case report. J Korean Med Sci. 2002 Feb;17(1):137-40.

[27] Ellen M. Chung. Pediatric Orbit Tumors and Tumorlike Lesions: Neuroepithelial Lesions of the Ocular Globe and Optic Nerve. RadioGraphics 2007; 27:1159-11

[28] Rubin CZ, Rosenfield NS, Abramson SJ, Abramson DH, Dunkel IJ The location and appearance of second malignancies in patients with bilateral retinoblastoma Sarcoma. 1997; 1(2):89-93

[29] Provenzale J M, Gururangan S and Klintworth G Trilateral Retinoblastoma: Clinical and Radiologic Progression. *AJR* 2004; 183:505-511

[30] Chang YW, Yoon HK, Shin HJ, Han BK. Suprasellar retinoblastoma in a 5-month-old girl. Pediatr Radiol. 2002 Dec; 32(12):869-71. Epub 2002 Jul 30.

[31] Bagley LJ, Hurst RW, Zimmerman RA, Shields JA, Shields CL, De Potter P. Imaging in the trilateral retinoblastoma syndrome . Neuroradiology. 1996 Feb; 38(2):166-70.

[32] Brenner D, Elliston C, Hall E et al. Estimated risks of radiation-induced fatal cancer from pediatric CT. AJR Am J Roentgenol 2001;176:289–296.

[33] Vasquez L M; Giuliari GP; HallidayW; Pavlin C J.; Gallie BL., ; Elise H. Eye Ultrasound Biomicroscopy in the Management of Retinoblastoma CME. CME Released: 01/14/2011; Valid for credit through 01/14/2012. Dept of Ophthalmology, University of Toronto, Canada

[34] Canturk S, Qaddoumi I, Khetan V, Ma Z, Furmanchuk A, Antoneli CB, Sultan I, Kebudi R, Sharma T, Rodriguez-Galindo C, Abramson DH, Chantada GL. Br J Ophthalmol. Survival of retinoblastoma in less-developed countries. Impact of socioeconomic and health-related indicators. 2010 Nov; 94(11):1432-6. Epub 2010 Aug 23.

[35] Honavar SG, Singh AD, Shields CL, et al. Post-enucleation prophylactic chemotherapy in high-risk retinoblastoma. Arch Ophthalmol 2002;120:923-931

[36] GÜndÜz K, MÜftÜoglu O, GÜnal I, Ünal E, Tacyildiz N · .Metastatic retinoblastoma : Clinical features, treatment, and prognosis .Ophthalmology. September 2006; 113(9): 1558-1566.

[37] Dunkel IJ, Aledo A, Kernan NA et al. Successful treatment of metastatic retinoblastoma. Cancer 2000; 89: 2117–2121.

[38] Kim J W, Kathpalia V, Dunkel I J Wong R K, Riedel E, Abramson DH. Orbital recurrence of retinoblastoma following enucleation .Br J Ophthalmol 2009; 93:463-467 doi:10.1136/bjo.2008.13845

[39] Bejjani GK, Donahue DJ, Selby D, Cogen PH, Packer R. Pediatr Neurosurg. 1996 Nov; 25(5):269-75..Association of a suprasellar mass and intraocular retinoblastoma: a variant of pineal trilateral retinoblastoma?

[40] Hernandez C, Brady LW, Shields JA, Shields CL, Depotter P, Karlson UL et al. External beam radiation for retinoblastoma: patterns of failure and proposal for treatment guidelines. Int J Radiat Oncol Biol phys. 1996; 35(1):125- 32

[41] Chintagumpala M, Chevez-Barrios P, Paysse EA, Plon SE, Hurwitz R Oncologist. 2007 . Oct;12(10):1237-46.

[42] Abramson DH, Melson MR, Dunkel IJ et al. Third (fourth and fifth) nonocular tumors in survivors of retinoblastoma. Ophthalmology. 2001; 108:1868-1876.

[43] Acquaviva A, Ciccolallo L, Rondelli R et al. Mortality from second tumour among long-term survivors of retinoblastoma: a retrospective analysis of the Italian retinoblastoma registry. Oncogene 2006; 25(38):5350-5357.

[44] Chantada GL, Gonzalez A, Fandino A, de Davila MT, Demirdjian G, Scopinaro M, Abramson D. Some clinical findings at presentation can predict high-risk pathology features in unilateral retinoblastoma. . J Pediatr Hematol Oncol 2009 May; 31(5):325-9.

[45] Uusitalo M S, Van Quill K R, Scott I U, Matthay K K, murray TG, Obrien JM. Evaluation of Chemoprophylaxis in Patients With Unilateral Retinoblastoma With High-Risk Features on Histopathologic Examination Arch ophthalmol 2001; 119:41-48

[46] Shields C L, Palamar Melis, Sharma P, Ramasubramanian A, Leahey A,Meadows A T, Shields J A. Retinoblastoma Regression Patterns Following Chemoreduction and Adjuvant Therapy in 557 Tumors. *Arch Ophthalmol.* 2009; 127(3):282-290.

[47] Wong FL, Boice JD Jr, Abramson DH et al. Cancer incidence after retinoblastoma. Radiation dose and sarcoma risk. JAMA 1997; 278:1262–7.

[48] Desjardins L, Chefchaouni MC, Lumbroso L et al. Functional Results After Treatment of Retinoblastoma. J AAPOS 2002; 6:108-11.

[49] Ibarra MS, O'Brien JM. Is screening for primitive neuroectodermal tumors in patients with unilateral retinoblastoma necessary? J AAPOS. 2000 Feb; 4(1):54-6.

[50] Demirci H, Shields C L, Meadows AT, Shields JA. Long-term Visual Outcome Following Chemoreduction for Retinoblastoma. *Arch Ophthalmol.* 2005; 123:1525-1530.

[51] Carol L. Shields, Jerry A. Shields. Diagnosis and Management of Retinoblastoma. Cancer Control. 2004; 11(5) © 2004 H. Lee Moffitt Cancer Center and Research Institute, Inc.

[52] Owoeye J FA, Afolayan EAO, Ademola-Popoola DS, Retinoblastoma - a clinico - pathological study in Ilorin, Nigeria. African Journal of Health Sciences, Vol. 13, No. 1-2, Jan-June, 2006, pp. 117-123

[53] Bekibele CO, Ayede AI, Asaolu OO, et al. Retinoblastoma: The challenges of management in Ibadan, Nigeria. J Pediatr Hematol Oncol 2009; 31: 552–555.

[54] Jenkinson H. Chemotherapy for retinoblastoma. Workshop: Retinoblastoma- 2011 and beyond. AAPOS2011. San Diego

[55] Tawansy KA, Samuel MA, Shammas M, Murphree AL. Vitreoretinal complications of retinoblastoma treatment. Retina. 2006 Sep; 26(7 Suppl):S47-52.

2

Second Malignancies in Retinoblastoma: The Real Problem

Basil K. Williams Jr. and Amy C. Schefler
Bascom Palmer Eye Institute, Department of Ophthalmology, University of Miami Miller School of Medicine
USA

1. Introduction

Retinoblastoma accounts for 6% of pediatric malignancies under the age of 5 years in the United States, (Broaddus et al., 2008) and epidemiological data suggest that the incidence is standard across populations (Kivelä, 2009). Despite its rarity, observations about the pathogenesis of this disease have enhanced our understanding of genetic cancer syndromes. Germinal or hereditary cases comprise approximately 40% of retinoblastoma cases, and all patients with the germinal *RB1* mutation are at risk for secondary malignancies. According to recent reports, some retinoblastoma patients exhibit varying degrees of mosaicism for the *RB1* mutation, allowing them to develop second primary malignancies in addition to those with standard hereditary retinoblastoma. These cancers occur in various anatomic locations such as the skull and long bones, soft tissues, skin, nasal cavity, brain, lung, and breast. The pattern of development and risk for these tumors are heavily influenced by the methods of treatment for retinoblastoma, which have shifted from enucleation to external-beam radiation to systemic chemotherapy with focal treatments. Investigations of the benefits of intra-arterial chemotherapy are ongoing with the hopes of reducing the morbidities associated with systemic therapy. Due to these improving treatment techniques, 10-year survival rates of primary retinoblastoma have been among the highest of all childhood cancers at greater than 92% in the United States and other developed countries since 1975 (Kaatsch, 2010; Linabery & Ross, 2008). Secondary malignancies have thus become an increasingly significant topic of interest as they are the leading cause of death of germinal retinoblastoma survivors in the United States.

2. History

The number of retinoblastoma survivors and their offspring increased during the mid-twentieth century as methods of detection and treatment regimens improved. This increased survival greatly enhanced insight into the pathology of retinoblastoma, including the identification of the somatic and germ-line mutation variants of sporadic retinoblastoma (Albert, 1987). Examination of the differences between unilateral and bilateral disease prompted the two-hit model of retinoblastoma by Knudson in 1971 (Knudson, 1971). This proposal led to the realization that hereditary patients carry a germinally inactivated *RB1* allele in all cells of the body before somatically suffering inactivation of the normal allele in a retinal cell or cells. Without the tumor suppressive activity of a functional pRB, these patients become susceptible to developing second nonocular cancers. Before the 1970s, the majority of new malignancies in survivors of retinoblastoma arose in the prior radiation fields, and could be labeled as radiation-induced neoplasias (Zimmerman, 1985). Secondary tumors arising from non-irradiated areas were initially reported by Jensen and Miller (Jensen & Miller, 1971) in 1971. In 1976 Abramson et al (Abramson, 1976) demonstrated the association of the risk of nonocular cancers with heritable retinoblastoma. Jakobiec et al. (Jakobiec et al., 1977) and Bader et al. (Bader et al., 1980) are responsible for the initial identification of trilateral retinoblastoma, the occurrence of a tumor in the pineal gland or parasellar region in addition to having hereditary retinoblastoma. Subsequently, the types of second cancers, risk factors for development of second cancers, and survival after development of second cancers have been extensively reviewed.

3. Epidemiology

Survivors of retinoblastoma who carry the *RB1* mutation are not at an increased risk of dying from any cause when compared to those who have not had retinoblastoma, with the exception of second non-ocular cancers. The incidence of secondary malignancies in germinal retinoblastoma survivors has been the topic of study in many reports, (Abramson et al., 2001; Eng et al., 1993; Fletcher et al., 2004; Kleinerman et al., 2005; MacCarthy et al., 2009; Marees et al., 2008; Moll et al., 1997; Wong et al., 1997; & Yu et al., 2009) but the variance of sample size and study design in these reports has made interpretation of the cumulative incidence difficult. Using reported cumulative risk rates from sizeable studies with appreciable long-term follow-up, incidence rates are approximately 0.5% to 1% per year. These are gross estimates used for comparison across studies (Fletcher et al., 2004). Long-term follow-up of a large cohort of 1,601 retinoblastoma survivors in the United States revealed a cumulative risk of a second cancer among hereditary patients of 36% at 50 years compared to only 5.7% in patients with sporadic retinoblastoma (Kleinerman et al., 2005). Similar results were observed in a large cohort of 1927 retinoblastoma survivors in Britain with a cumulative overall incidence of second cancer among hereditary patients of 43% at 50 years compared to only 4.9% in nonhereditary retinoblastoma survivors (MacCarthy et al., 2009).

Epidemiologic evidence has indicated that incidence rates may vary based on the treatment received by the patient and the age at which it is received. It has been well documented that patients who were irradiated for retinoblastoma have a higher incidence of secondary malignancies than those who were not irradiated. Furthermore, 50% of patients who developed retinoblastoma within the first month of life and were treated with radiotherapy developed second cancers by 24 years of age (Abramson et al., 2002a). The incidence of retinoblastoma has remained stable over the last 30 years in the United States, (Broaddus et al., 2008) but the cumulative incidence of new cancers has declined as the dosage and use of radiotherapy continues to decrease (Kleinerman et al., 2005). As new and better therapies are developed this trend is likely to continue.

4. Types of second tumors

4.1 Benign

In a survey of 898 retinoblastoma survivors, Li et al. (Li et al., 1997) reported a surprising number of lipomas in patients with this hereditary disease. Rieder et al. (Rieder et al., 1998) futher promoted the idea that a predisposing *RB1* gene mutation may play a role in the development of lipomas in retinoblastoma patients, by demonstrating the recurrent loss of the same *RB1* allele in two different lipomas in the same patient. Others have reported a genetic linkage between a specific *RB1* mutation and the development of multiple lipomas, postulating that there is a linked polymorphic allele which acts as a modifying factor by affecting expression of the *RB1* gene mutation (Genuardi et al., 2001). These lipomas, when found in hereditary retinoblastoma patients, are preferentially located on the face, neck, shoulders, and upper chest (Genuardi et al., 2001). Li et al. (Li et al., 1997) additionally, found twice as many patients with hereditary retinoblastoma and lipomas developed secondary malignancies when compared to those without lipomas. These results suggest that the presence of lipomas may indicate an elevated second cancer risk and that certain germline mutations in the *RB1* gene may predispose the patient to both lipomas and secondary tumors. This finding may have future implications on follow up and screening of retinoblastoma survivors for second malignancies.

4.2 Malignant

The most common second malignancies appear to be closely related to the initial method of treatment for retinoblastoma. In the United States and the Netherlands, where external beam radiation was commonly used as primary therapy, osteosarcomas of the skull and long bones, soft tissue sarcomas, cutaneous melanomas, brain tumors including trilateral retinoblastoma, tumors of the nasal cavity, Hodgkin's disease, lung cancer, and breast cancer predominate (Kleinerman et al., 2005; MacCarthy et al., 2009; Marees et al., 2008; Wong et al., 1997). In Britain, where the majority of retinoblastoma survivors did not undergo external beam radiation, epithelial cancers were more common, especially as follow-up extended into the seventh decade (Fletcher et al., 2004). As trends in treatment continue to change and the length of follow-up continues to increase, the rate of bone and soft tissue cancer development may decline while the rate of epithelial cancers are likely to increase.

Studies on the development of additional tumors (third, fourth and fifth) in survivors of retinoblastoma and second malignancies have been performed, although without consistent results (Abramson et al., 2001, Marees et al., 2010). Epidemiologically, Abramson et al. (Abramson et al., 2001) demonstrated an incidence rate of approximately 2% per year from the time of diagnosis of the second malignancy. Marees et al. (Marees et al., 2010) reported an 8-fold increase in the risk for a third primary neoplasm compared to the general population. The latency period decreases as each additional cancer is diagnosed. Historically, male retinoblastoma survivors were reported to have a higher incidence of third malignancies, primarily because females had an increased overall mortality rate from second malignancies (Abramson et al., 2001; Eng et al., 1993). More recent studies, however, have no longer identified an increase in female mortality from second malignancies (Marees et al., 2009; Yu et al., 2009). Abramson et al. (Abramson et al., 2001) reported a predictable pattern for third, fourth, and fifth malignancy development based on location of the second tumor. In that study, patients with second malignancies of the skin or skull were more likely to develop an additional tumor in the skin and skull, respectively. Marees et al. (Marees et al., 2010) did not find this predictable pattern in a Dutch cohort.

4.3 Trilateral retinoblastoma

Trilateral retinoblastoma is a well-recognized syndrome that consists of unilateral or bilateral retinoblastoma associated with an intracranial primitive neuroectodermal tumor. The intracranial mass is often located in the pineal region, but may also be a suprasellar or parasellar tumor. A specific subset of patients are more likely to develop these lesions including those with a family history of retinoblastoma, bilateral disease, diagnosis within the first 6 months of life, and prior treatment with external beam radiation. Reviews of published cases of trilateral retinoblastoma from 1966 through 1998 and 1977 through 1997 demonstrated a poor prognosis with a median survival of 6 to 9 months (Kivelä, 1999, Paulino, 1999). More recently, a small series from Brazil corroborated the dismal prognosis by reporting a median survival of 10 months (Antoneli et al., 2007). As such, these tumors are the most frequent cause of death in retinoblastoma survivors between the ages of 5 to 10 years (Blach et al., 1994). However, promising new studies indicate that treatment of trilateral retinoblastoma with intensive chemotherapy may offer an improved prognosis (Dimaras et al., 2011; Dunkel et al., 2009).

The incidence of trilateral retinoblastoma has decreased recently, but the underlying cause for this shift remains controversial. Shields et al. (Shields et al., 2001) suggested that chemoreduction therapy may reduce the incidence of pineoblastoma. Of the 99 at risk patients treated with chemoreduction in that study, none developed pineoblastoma. However, 1 of 18 (5.5%) at risk patients not treated with chemoreduction developed trilateral retinoblastoma, which is consistent with the rate of development in other published series. None of the patients in the chemoreduction group were treated with radiotherapy, prompting some to suggest that the declining incidence of pineoblastomas may be due to the declining use of external-beam radiation therapy (Moll et al., 2002). An analysis of the published literature by Woo et al. in 2010 reported an approximately equal number of pinealomas in irradiated patients and those who were not irradiated, suggesting that radiation therapy may not play as significant a role in trilateral retinoblastoma as previously suspected (Woo & Harbour, 2010). Additional studies are needed to elucidate the relationship between chemoreduction and trilateral retinoblastoma.

It is important to note that the classification of these tumors as a second malignancy as opposed to a variant of the primary tumor is controversial. They often cannot be differentiated from retinoblastoma histologically and have occasionally been documented to occur prior to the development of ocular manifestations in some patients (Jurkiewicz et al., 2009; Moll et al., 2001) For these reasons, some studies have not included trilateral retinoblastoma as a second malignancy, but the classification has varied over the years causing some discrepancy in the literature.

4.4 Independent second non-ocular retinoblastoma

Soh et al. (Soh et al., 2011) reported a case of an independent retinoblastoma located in the ovary of a bilateral ophthalmic retinoblastoma survivor. Eighteen years after radiation of the right eye and enucleation of the left eye, the patient was found to have a large left ovarian tumor involving the fallopian tube, mesentery, and lymph nodes. Histologically, the concurrent presence of Homer Wright and Flexner-Wintersteiner rosettes confirmed the identification as retinoblastoma. Additionally, molecular analysis demonstrated mutations of both *RB1* alleles, but a different pattern of post-*RB1* mutational events from the tumors in the eye in this patient. This difference suggests that the ovarian tumor was of a separate clonal origin from the original eye tumor. While the reasons for retinoblastoma arising ectopically in ovarian tissue are unclear, primitive neuroectodermal tumors (trilateral retinoblastoma) have been documented as second malignancies in survivors of retinoblastoma.

5. Risk factors for the development of second malignancies

5.1 Rb1 mutation

Studies have indicated that all retinoblastoma survivors who develop second malignancies carry the germinal *RB1* mutation, which inactivates the tumor suppressor gene that is expressed in all adult tissues. The protein encoded by *RB1* functions in multiple cellular processes including proliferation, DNA replication, DNA repair, and cell-cycle checkpoint control. The timing of initiation of the expression of pRB varies in each cell type, rendering patients who carry the *RB1* mutation at risk of developing malignancies in nonocular tissues.

Patients who carry the germ-line *RB1* mutation (approximately 40% of total retinoblastoma patients) have bilateral disease in up to 85% of cases. The remaining 15%, with unilateral disease, are also at increased risk for developing second cancers (Abramson et al., 2001). Patients with unilateral disease who are at high risk for carrying the germinal mutation, and therefore at increased risk for developing a second malignancy, have been identified by clinical observation. They consist of patients with a family history of retinoblastoma, patients diagnosed within the first 6 months of life, and patients with multifocal disease. Advances in mutation analysis have shown that mosaic *RB1* mutations are more common than previously thought, accounting for at least 5.5 and 3.8% of bilateral and unilateral cases, respectively (Rushlow et al., 2009). This has implications for genetic counseling conversations, as many patients likely fall on a spectrum of risk for the development of second cancers.

Long-term studies of retinoblastoma survivors in the Netherlands demonstrated a 20.4-fold increase in second malignancy compared with the general population (Marees et al. 2008). There was not a significant difference in risk of second malignancies between nonhereditary survivors and the general population.

5.2 Retinoma

Retinoma or retinocytoma is a rare intraocular malignancy that appears to be a benign variant of retinoblastoma. These lesions display inactivations of both RB1 allelles and represent a step towards retinoblastoma development (Dimaras et al., 2008; Sampieri et al., 2008). At least 6 cases of patients with a retinoma and a second primary tumor have been published in the literature, indicating there is likely an increased risk of second malignancies in this population (Korswagen et al., 2004).

5.3 External beam radiation therapy

As the primary treatment method for retinoblastoma through much of the latter half of the 20th century, external beam radiation and its effects on second primary malignancies have been extensively studied. Numerous studies of varying designs have reported a clear increase in second nonocular malignancies in patients who have undergone external beam radiation (Aerts et al., 2004; Marees et al., 2008; Moll et al., 2001, Wong et al., 1997). Kleinerman et al. (Kleinerman et al., 2005) reported that the cumulative risk of a second cancer among irradiated hereditary patients was 38% at 50 years compared to 21% among non-irradiated hereditary patients. Due to the proximity to the radiation field and consequent radiation exposure, there is an increase in head and neck tumors and brain tumors in retinoblastoma patients who have been previously irradiated (Abramson, 2005; Aerts et al., 2004; Kleinerman et al., 2005; Marees et al., 2009). More recent studies with longer follow-up have also demonstrated an increased risk of epithelial neoplasms in this population, but these may not be attributed to the effects of radiation (Marees et al., 2008). In addition to affecting the location of subsequent tumor development, radiation exposure appears to cause an earlier onset of second malignancies (Abramson, 2005; Chauveinc et al., 2001). Mortality has also been reported to occur earlier as irradiated hereditary retinoblastoma patients died sooner than their non-irradiated counterparts with a median age of death of 20.5 years and 40 years, respectively (Yu et al., 2009). The dose-dependent relationship of radiation administration and the development of second malignancies was established over 40 years ago, (Sagerman et al., 1969) and more recent studies have confirmed this analysis (Kleinerman et al., 2005; Wong et al., 1997). The age at which radiation therapy is administered seems to influence the incidence of second tumor development, as patients treated under the age of 1 year were twice as likely to develop a second malignancy than those radiated after the age of 1 year (Abramson & Frank, 1998). In fact, patients treated with radiation therapy after the first year of life do not seem to have an increased risk of second tumor development when compared to those who were never irradiated. Because of these effects and advancements in the use of chemotherapy, use of external beam radiation therapy has decreased significantly over the last decade. Moreover, when it is used, there is a focus on minimizing the radiation dose and limiting the field of radiation as much as possible (Chan et al., 2009; Munier et al., 2008).

5.4 Preventable risk factors

5.4.1 Sun exposure

The degree of sunlight exposure has not been directly correlated to the development of cutaneous melanoma specifically in survivors of retinoblastoma. However, the known association between ultraviolet radiation and cutaneous melanoma in the general population combined with the increased incidence of cutaneous melanomas in retinoblastoma survivors is sufficient evidence to recommend avoidance of sunlight (Trappey et al., 2010).

5.4.2 Smoking

Retinoblastoma survivors should be aggressively counseled to refrain from smoking as multiple studies have indicated an excess incidence of lung cancer and risk of death from lung cancer in relatives of retinoblastoma patients who are carriers of the *RB1* gene mutation (Sanders et al., 1989; Strong et al., 1984). The elevated risk of lung cancer and the greater risk of death from lung cancer were also demonstrated in survivors of hereditary retinoblastoma (Fletcher et al., 2004; Kleinerman et al., 2000; Marees et al., 2008; Yu et al., 2009). Moreover, the risk of death in the hereditary survivor population was sevenfold greater than in the general population (Fletcher et al., 2004). In 2000, Kleinerman et al. (Kleinerman et al., 2000) demonstrated similar smoking rates between the general population and survivors of both hereditary and nonhereditary retinoblastoma. However more recently, Foster et al. (Foster et al., 2006) reported that hereditary survivors actually smoked significantly less than nonhereditary survivors and less than the general United States population. While smoking rates in retinoblastoma survivors appear to be improving, it is imperative that physicians encourage survivors to quit or abstain from smoking. Counseling on abstinence for smoking may also have an effect on the development of bladder cancer in this population, as an increased risk for bladder cancer in retinoblastoma survivors has been demonstrated when compared with the general population (Frobisher et al., 2010; Kleinerman et al., 2005; Marees et al., 2008). While smoking was not specifically associated with bladder cancers in this cohort, it has been shown to be the most important environmental risk factor in the general population (Hirao et al., 2009).

5.4.3 CT scans

The risk of carcinogenesis secondary to radiation exposure from computed tomography (CT) has become the focus of increased investigation over the last few decades. Epidemiological data suggests that there is a larger attributable lifetime cancer mortality risk for children undergoing radiation when compared to adults (Brenner et al., 2001; Mills et al., 2006). In fact, radiation doses above 50 millisieverts (mSv) in children and 100 mSv in adults, which can be attained with repeated imaging, increases the risk for cancer (Pauwels & Bourguignon, 2011). The effective dose of CT scans vary from approximately 2 mSv for a head CT scan to approximately 20mSv for a CT-based coronary angiography study (Pauwels & Bourguignon, 2011). With the amount of scans required for appropriate cancer surveillance, retinoblastoma survivors will likely reach doses that increase the risk of cancer. Considering the increased risk of developing radiation-induced cancers in patients with a germinal *RB1* mutation and the increased sensitivity to the carcinogenic effects of radiation in children, this cohort should avoid all forms of unnecessary radiation. For these reasons, some radiologists are recommending the avoidance of ionizing radiation altogether in retinoblastoma survivors and other populations at risk for secondary cancers (Vazquez et al., 2003).

5.5 Controversial risk factors

5.5.1 Chemotherapy

Chemotherapy has been part of the treatment regimen for retinoblastoma since the 1950s (Reese et al., 1954). Triethylene melamine was the chemotherapeutic agent of choice, often in conjunction with radiotherapy, throughout the 1950s and 1960s and was shown to increase the development of second tumors outside the field of radiation (Schlienger et al., 2004). In the 1990s, many centers began to shift from radiation towards systemic chemotherapy with an increasing focus on intra-arterial chemotherapy over the last 5 years. Because of the recent shift in management, there are not many long-term studies examining the effects on second primary neoplasms. As a result, the role of chemotherapy in the development of second cancers remains controversial. Most often current chemotherapy regimens consist of vincristine, carboplatin, and an epipodophyllotoxin, either etoposide or tenoposide.

Cyclosporine has been used in addition to this combination to decrease the development of multidrug resistance. Both platinum-based drugs and topoisomerase inhibitors have been reported to increase the risk of second tumors in other primary malignancies (Hijiya et al., 2009; Klein et al., 2003; Travis et al., 1999). Some studies have reported the development of acute myelogenous leukemia and secondary leukemia in retinoblastoma survivors treated with epipodophyllotoxins and alkylating agents, respectively (Gallegos-Castorena et al., 2002; Gombos et al., 2007; Nishimura et al., 2001; Weintraub et al., 2007). In a study of 187 patients with hereditary retinoblastoma treated with carboplatin, vincristine +/- etoposide, 6 patients developed second malignancies (Turaka et al., 2011). Only 1 of these 6 developed acute myelogenous leukemia, and that patient was also treated with external beam radiation. While this study had a relatively short follow-up, the patients were followed for longer than the average latency for development of chemotherapy-related acute myelogenous leukemia. Considering this, the authors suggest that the low incidence of therapy-based leukemia in this study is reassuring. With the increased use of intra-arterial chemotherapy, direct administration via the ophthalmic artery, over the last 5 to 6 years, the systemic exposure to chemotherapy is significantly reduced. This may reduce the carcinogenic risk of chemotherapy in this population. Further studies are needed to elucidate the relationship between both intra-arterial and systemic chemotherapy and second malignant neoplasms.

5.5.2 Growth hormone

Growth hormone (GH), a treatment often administered to pediatric oncology survivors, has mitogenic and proliferogenic properties that may theoretically lead to disease recurrence or increased development of secondary neoplasms. Sklar et al. (Sklar et al., 2002) reported that treatment with GH for pediatric cancer patients may increase the risk of a secondary solid tumor, although the overall increased risk was driven largely by a small subgroup of acute leukemia survivors. A follow-up study by Ergun-Longmire et al. (Ergun-Longmire et al., 2006) concurred with the increased risk of secondary neoplasms but suggested that the risk appears to diminish with increasing length of follow-up. In 2002, Abramson et al. (Abramson et al., 2002b) reported a case of a metastatic germinal retinoblastoma survivor treated with GH who subsequently developed an osteogenic sarcoma. A more recent study by Bell et al. (Bell et al., 2009) reported 4.6 second tumor cases per 1000 patient-years of GH exposure. Leukemia was the most common primary malignancy associated with secondary tumors after growth hormone, but proportionately, retinoblastoma had a higher frequency of neoplasms. Five of the sixteen patients with retinoblastoma as the primary neoplasm developed secondary cancers. Of these, 4 were previously treated with radiation therapy, and only 3 occurred in patients with bilateral retinoblastoma. While these findings are of some concern, larger studies examining the risk of secondary cancers in retinoblastoma survivors need to be performed to derive conclusive results.

6. Survival

Although the survival rates of primary retinoblastoma are continually improving, the outcome of second malignancies does not appear to be improving with time. Reulen et al. (Reulen et al., 2010) examined the long-term cause-specific mortality among 18,000 survivors of childhood cancer in Britain, and reported a standardized mortality ratio of 24.7

Study	Location	Period	Number of Hereditary Rb Patients	Number of SMN	Cumulative Risk of SMN Development	Number of Sporadic Rb Patients	Number of SMN	Cumulative Risk of SMN Development	Number of Total Rb Patients	Number of SMN	Cumulative Risk of SMN Development
Acquaviva et al., 2006°	Italy	1923-2003	408	31		703	7		1111	38	
Araki et al. 2011	Japan	1964-2007	372		33.8% at 40 years after diagnosis	382		1% at 30 years after diagnosis	754	21	19.1% at 40 years after treatment*
Fletcher et al., 2004§	United Kingdom	?	144		68.8% at 84 years of age						
Kleinerman et al., 2005	United States	1914-1984	963	260	36% at 50 years after diagnosis	638	17	5.69% at 50 years after diagnosis	1601	277	
MacCarthy et al., 2009	United Kingdom	1951-2004	809	102	48.3% at 50 years after diagnosis*	1118	13	4.9% at 50 years after diagnosis*	1927	115	
Marees et al., 2008	Netherlands	1945-2005	298	62	28% at 40 years after diagnosis	370	12	1.44% at 40 years after diagnosis	668	74	

Abbreviation: Rb, retinoblastoma; SMN, secondary malignant neoplasm. §Included hereditary patients only. ° Included pineoblastoma as a secondary malignancy. *Adjusted for competing risk of death.

Table 1. Reported Risk of Second Nonocular Cancers in Retinoblastoma Survivors

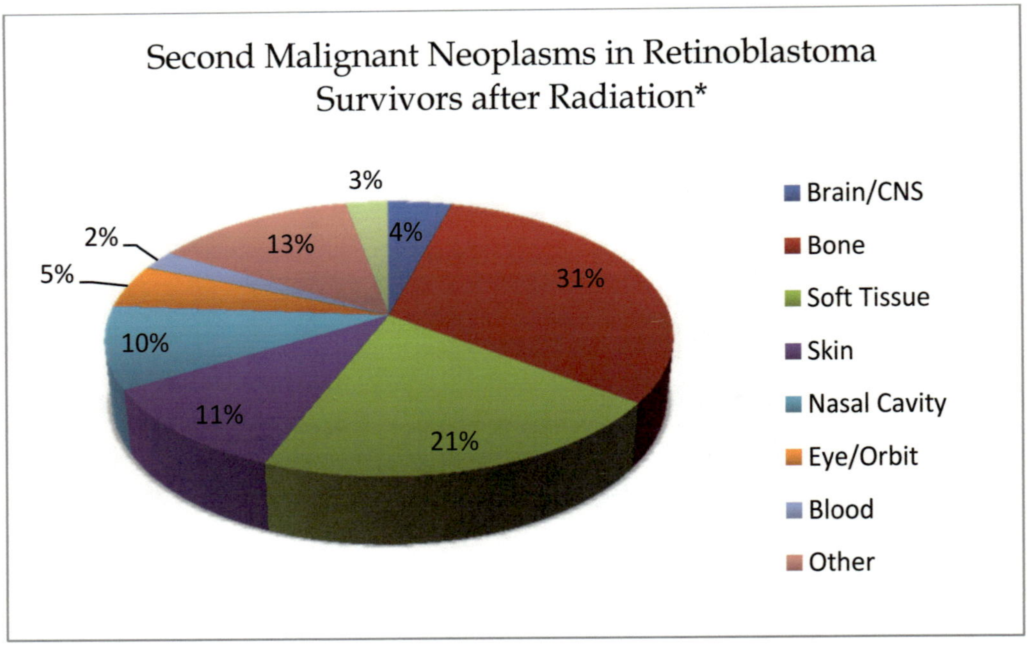

*Radiation included external beam radiation and brachytherapy in all studies except Marees et al., 2008, which did not include brachytherapy as radiation.

Fig. 1. Pie chart demonstrating the histologic type of reported second malignant neoplasms in patients treated with radiation (Acquaviva et al., 2006; Aerts et al., 2004; Kleinerman et al., 2005; Marees et al., 2008; & Turaka et al., 2011). Some of these patients may have been treated with chemotherapy, but this information was not identified in all of the studies.

due to second cancer deaths for hereditary retinoblastoma. In the Netherlands, Marees et al. (Marees et al., 2009) reported an almost 13-fold increase of second malignancy death comparing hereditary retinoblastoma survivors to the general population. As previously stated, outcome is particularly grim in patients with trilateral retinoblastoma who have a median survival of less than 12 months. A recent long-term study of 1854 retinoblastoma survivors from the United States reported a cause-specific cumulative mortality from subsequent malignant neoplasms of 26% in hereditary survivors and 1% for nonhereditary survivors 50 years after retinoblastoma diagnosis (Yu et al., 2009). An excess in overall cancer mortality has also been reported in unilateral sporadic retinoblastoma survivors, likely because some of these patients are unilaterally affected *RB1* mutation carriers (Acquaviva et al., 2006; Yu et al., 2009). While earlier studies reported a higher mortality from second tumors in females, more recent studies have indicated an equivalent mortality in males and females.

7. Screening

Screening practices for secondary tumors in retinoblastoma survivors have not been extensively studied and no universal protocol has been determined to date. Sheen et al. (Sheen et al., 2008) examined the cancer screening behavior in 875 retinoblastoma survivors. The rates of patients ≥40 years who underwent a mammogram within the past 2 years and

≥18 years who underwent a Papanicolau smear within the past 3 years were comparable between retinoblastoma survivors, other childhood cancer survivors who had received chest or mantle irradiation, and the general US population. Hereditary survivors were 3 times more likely to undergo an MRI or CT scan as a screening tool for second cancers. Neuroimaging with MRI has been recommended as the primary imaging modality, particularly in young retinoblastoma survivors, because of the increased risk for second malignancies with repeated exposure to ionizing radiation (ie. CT scans). However, a prospective study of routine screening with MRI performed in 226 retinoblastoma patients did not yield improved outcomes in patients who developed trilateral retinoblastoma (Duncan et al., 2001).

8. Conclusion

As treatment methods for retinoblastoma continue to evolve, the type and distribution of second non-ocular malignancies will continue to change. External beam radiation, once the mainstay of primary retinoblastoma management, increases the incidence of and mortality from second neoplasms, especially in the head and neck area. With an increased use of chemotherapy and longer duration of follow-up, malignancies of epithelial origin may become more common in this cohort. The potential for an increase in therapy-related leukemia is present with the use of chemotherapy, but additional long-term studies are required to assess the validity of this relationship. Survivors of retinoblastoma, particularly patients carrying a germinal *RB1* mutation or who have a retinoma, should undergo lifelong surveillance for second primary tumors. They should also avoid smoking, damaging exposure to sunlight, and ionizing radiation when possible.

9. References

Abramson, D.H., Ellsworth, R.M., & Zimmerman, L.E. (1976). Nonocular cancer in retinoblastoma survivors. *Trans Sect Ophthalmol Am Acad Ophthalmol Otolaryngol*, Vol.81, No.3 Pt.1, (May-Jun 1976), pp. 454-457

Abramson, D.H., & Frank, C.M. (1998). Second nonocular tumors in survivors of bilateral retinoblastoma: a possible age effect on radiation-related risk. *Ophthalmology*, Vol.105, No.4, (Apr 1998), pp. 573-579, ISSN 0161-6420

Abramson, D.H., Melson, M.R., Dunkel, I.J., & Frank, C.M. (2001). Third (fourth and fifth) nonocular tumors in survivors of retinoblastoma. *Ophthalmology*, Vol.108, No.10, (Oct 2001), pp. 1868-1876, ISSN 0161-6420

Abramson, D.H., Du, T.T., & Beaverson, K.L. (2002a). (Neonatal) retinoblastoma in the first month of life. *Arch Ophthalmol*, Vol.120, No.6, (Jun 2002), pp. 738-742, ISSN 0003-9950

Abramson, D.H., Lee, T.C., & Driscoll, C. (2002b). Osteogenic sarcoma in a survivor of metastatic germline retinoblastoma: the possible influence of human growth hormone. *J Pediatr Ophthalmol Strabismus*, Vol.39, No.6, (Nov-Dec 2002), pp. 347-348, ISSN 0191-3913

Abramson, D.H. (2005). Retinoblastoma in the 20th century: past success and future challenges the Weisenfeld lecture. *Invest Ophthalmol Vis Sci*, Vol.46, No.8, (Aug 2005), pp. 2683-2691, ISSN 0146-0404

Acquaviva, A., Ciccolallo, L., Rondelli, R., et al. (2006). Mortality from second tumour among long-term survivors of retinoblastoma: a retrospective analysis of the Italian retinoblastoma registry. *Oncogene*, Vol.25, No.38, (Aug 2006), pp. 5350-5357, ISSN 0950-9232

Aerts, I., Pacquement, H., Doz, F., et al. (2004). Outcome of second malignancies after retinoblastoma: a retrospective analysis of 25 patients treated at the Institut Curie. *Eur J Cancer*, Vol.40, No.10, (Jul 2004), pp. 1522-1529, ISSN 0959-8049

Albert, D.M. (1987). Historic review of retinoblastoma. *Ophthalmology*, Vol.94, No.6, (Jun 1987), pp. 654-662, ISSN 0161-6420

Antoneli, C.B., Ribeiro Kde, C., Sakamoto, L.H., et al. (2007). Trilateral retinoblastoma. *Pediatr Blood Cancer*, Vol.48, No.3, (Mar 2007), pp. 306-310, ISSN 1545-5009

Araki, Y., Matsuyama, Y., Kobayashi, Y., et al. (2010). Secondary neoplasms after retinoblastoma treatment: retrospective cohort study of 754 patients in Japan. *Jpn J Clin Oncol*, Vol.41, No.3, (Mar 2011), pp373-379, ISSN 0368-2811

Bader, J.L., Miller, R.W., Meadows, A.T., et al. (1980). Trilateral retinoblastoma. *Lancet*, Vol.2, No.8194, (Sep 1980), pp. 582-583, ISSN 0140-6736

Bell, J., Parker, K.L., Swinford, R.D., et al. (2009). Long-term safety of recombinant human growth hormone in children. *J Clin Endocrinol Metab*, Vol.95, No.1, (Jan 2010), pp. 167-177, ISSN 0021-972X

Blach, L.E., McCormick, B., Abramson, D.H., & Ellsworth, R.M. (1994). Trilateral retinoblastoma--incidence and outcome: a decade of experience. *Int J Radiat Oncol Biol Phys*, Vol.29, No.4, (Jul 1994), pp. 729-733

Brenner, D., Elliston, C., Hall, E., & Berdon, W. (2001). Estimated risks of radiation-induced fatal cancer from pediatric CT. *AJR Am J Roentgenol*, Vol.176, No.2, (Feb 2001), pp. 289-296, ISSN 0360-3016

Broaddus, E., Topham, A., & Singh, A.D. (2008). Incidence of retinoblastoma in the USA: 1975-2004. *Br J Ophthalmol*, Vol.93, No.1, (Jan 2009), pp. 21-23, ISSN 0007-1161

Chan, M.P., Hungerford, J.L., Kingston, J.E., & Plowman, P.N. (2009). Salvage external beam radiotherapy after failed primary chemotherapy for bilateral retinoblastoma: rate of eye and vision preservation. *Br J Ophthalmol*, Vol.93, No.7, (Jul 2009), pp. 891-894, ISSN 0007-1161

Chauveinc, L., Mosseri, V., Quintana, E., et al. (2001). Osteosarcoma following retinoblastoma: age at onset and latency period. *Ophthalmic Genet*, Vol.22, No.2, (Jun 2001), pp. 77-88, ISSN 1381-6810

Dimaras, H., Khetan, V., Halliday, W., et al. (2008). Loss of RB1 induces non-proliferative retinoma: increasing genomic instability correlates with progression to retinoblastoma. *Hum Mol Genet*, Vol.17, No.10, (May 2008), pp. 1363-1372, ISSN 0964-6906

Dimaras, H., Héon, E., Doyle, J., et al. (2011). Multifaceted chemotherapy for trilateral retinoblastoma. *Arch Ophthalmol*, Vol.129, No.3, (Mar 2011), pp. 362-365, ISSN 0003-9950

Duncan, J.L., Scott, I.U., Murray, T.G., et al. (2001). Routine neuroimaging in retinoblastoma for the detection of intracranial tumors. *Arch Ophthalmol*, Vol.119, No.3, (Mar 2001), pp. 450-452, ISSN 0003-9950

Dunkel, I.J., Jubran, R.F., Gururangan, S., et al. (2010). Trilateral retinoblastoma: potentially curable with intensive chemotherapy. *Pediatr Blood Cancer*, Vol.54, No.3, (Mar 2010), pp. 384-387, ISSN 1545-5009

Eng, C., Li, F.P., Abramson, D.H., et al. (1993). Mortality from second tumors among long-term survivors of retinoblastoma. *J Natl Cancer Inst*, Vol.85, No.14, (Jul 1993), pp. 1121-1128, ISSN 0027-8874

Ergun-Longmire, B., Mertens, A.C., Mitby, P., et al. (2006). Growth hormone treatment and risk of second neoplasms in the childhood cancer survivor. *J Clin Endocrinol Metab*, Vol.91, No.9, (Sep 2006), pp. 3494-3498, ISSN 0021-972X

Fletcher, O., Easton, D., Anderson, K., et al. (2004). Lifetime risks of common cancers among retinoblastoma survivors. *J Natl Cancer Inst*, Vol.96, No.5, (Mar 2004), pp. 357-363, ISSN 0027-8874

Foster, M.C., Kleinerman, R.A., Abramson, D., et al. (2006). Tobacco use in adult long-term survivors of retinoblastoma. *Cancer Epidemiol Biomarkers Prev*, Vol.15, No.8, (Aug 2006), pp. 1464-1468, ISSN 1055-9965

Frobisher, C., Gurung, P.M., Leiper, A., et al. (2010). Risk of bladder tumours after childhood cancer: the British Childhood Cancer Survivor Study. *BJU Int*, Vol.106, No.7, (Oct 2010), pp. 1060-1069, ISSN 1464-4096

Gallegos-Castorena, S., Medina-Sansón, A., González-Montalvo, P., et al. (2002). Letter to the editor: acute myeloid leukemia in a patient surviving retinoblastoma. *Med Pediatr Oncol*, Vol.38, No.6, (Jun 2002), pp. 450, ISSN 0098-1532

Genuardi, M., Klutz, M., Devriendt, K., et al. (2001). Multiple lipomas linked to an RB1 gene mutation in a large pedigree with low penetrance retinoblastoma. *Eur J Hum Genet*, Vol.9, No.9, (Sep 2001), pp. 690-694, ISSN 1018-4813

Gombos, D.S., Hungerford, J., Abramson, D.H., et al. (2007). Secondary acute myelogenous leukemia in patients with retinoblastoma: is chemotherapy a factor? *Ophthalmology*, Vol.114, No.7, (Jul 2007), pp. 1378-1383, ISSN 0161-6420

Hijiya, N., Ness, K.K., Ribeiro, R.C., & Hudson, M.M. (2009). Acute leukemia as a secondary malignancy in children and adolescents: current findings and issues. *Cancer*, Vol.115, No.1, (Jan 2009), pp. 23-35, ISSN 0008-543X

Hirao, Y., Kim, W.J., & Fujimoto, K. (2009). Environmental factors promoting bladder cancer. *Curr Opin Urol*, Vol.19, No.5, (Sep 2009), pp. 494-499, ISSN 0963-0643

Jakobiec, F.A., Tso, M.O., Zimmerman, L.E., & Danis, P. (1977). Retinoblastoma and intracranial malignancy. *Cancer*, Vol.39, No.5, (May 1977), pp. 2048-2058, ISSN 0008-543X

Jensen, R.D., & Miller, R.W. (1971). Retinoblastoma: epidemiologic characteristics. *N Engl J Med*, Vol.285, No.6, (Aug 1971), pp. 307-311, ISSN 0028-4793

Jurkiewicz, E., Pakuła-Kościesza, I., Rutynowska, O., & Nowak, K. (2009). Trilateral retinoblastoma: an institutional experience and review of the literature. *Childs Nerv Syst*, Vol.26, No.1, (Jan 2010), pp. 129-132, ISSN 1433-0350

Kaatsch, P. (2010). Epidemiology of childhood cancer. *Cancer Treat Rev*, Vol.36, No.4, (Jun 2010), pp. 277-285, ISSN 0305-7372

Klein, G., Michaelis, J., Spix, C., et al. (2003). Second malignant neoplasms after treatment of childhood cancer. *Eur J Cancer*, Vol.39, No.6, (Apr 2003), pp. 808-817, ISSN 0959-8049

Kleinerman, R.A., Tucker, M.A., Tarone, R.E., et al. (2005). Risk of new cancers after radiotherapy in long-term survivors of retinoblastoma: an extended follow-up. *J Clin Oncol*, Vol.23, No.10, (Apr 2005), pp. 2272-2279, ISSN 0732-183X

Kivelä, T. (1999). Trilateral retinoblastoma: a meta-analysis of hereditary retinoblastoma associated with primary ectopic intracranial retinoblastoma. *J Clin Oncol*, Vol.17, No.6, (Jun 1999), pp. 1829-1837, ISSN 0732-183X

Kivelä, T. (2009). The epidemiological challenge of the most frequent eye cancer: retinoblastoma, an issue of birth and death. *Br J Ophthalmol*, Vol.93, No.9, (Sep 2009), pp. 1129-1131, ISSN 0007-1161

Knudson, A.G. Jr. (1971). Mutation and cancer: statistical study of retinoblastoma. *Proc Natl Acad Sci U S A*, Vol.68, No.4, (Apr 1971), pp. 820-823, ISSN 0027-8424

Korswagen, L.A., Moll, A.C., Imhof, S.M., & Schouten-van Meeteren, A.Y. (2004). A second primary tumor in a patient with retinoma. *Ophthalmic Genet*, Vol.25, No.1, (Mar 2004), pp. 45-48, ISSN 1381-6810

Li, F.P., Abramson, D.H., Tarone, R.E., et al. (1997). Hereditary retinoblastoma, lipoma, and second primary cancers. *J Natl Cancer Inst*, Vol.89, No.1, (Jan 1997), pp. 83-84, ISSN 0027-8874

Linabery, A.M., & Ross, J.A. (2008). Childhood and adolescent cancer survival in the US by race and ethnicity for the diagnostic period 1975-1999. *Cancer*, Vol.113, No.9, (Nov 2008), pp. 2575-2596, ISSN 0008-543X

MacCarthy, A., Bayne, A.M., Draper, G.J., et al. (2009). Non-ocular tumours following retinoblastoma in Great Britain 1951 to 2004. *Br J Ophthalmol*, Vol.93, No.9, (2009), pp. 1159-1162, ISSN 0007-1161

Marees, T., Moll, A.C., Imhof, S.M., et al. (2008). Risk of second malignancies in survivors of retinoblastoma: more than 40 years of follow-up. *J Natl Cancer Inst*, Vol.100, No.24, (Dec 2008), pp. 1771-1779, ISSN 0027-8874

Marees, T., van Leeuwen, F.E., de Boer, M.R., et al. (2009). Cancer mortality in long-term survivors of retinoblastoma. *Eur J Cancer*, Vol.45, No.18, (Dec 2009), pp. 3245-3253, ISSN 0959-8049

Marees, T., van Leeuwen, F.E., Schaapveld, M., et al. (2010). Risk of third malignancies and death after a second malignancy in retinoblastoma survivors. *Eur J Cancer*, Vol.46, No.11, (Jul 2010), pp. 2052-2058, ISSN 0959-8049

Mills, D.M., Tsai, S., Meyer, D.R., & Belden, C. (2006). Pediatric ophthalmic computed tomographic scanning and associated cancer risk. *Am J Ophthalmol*, Vol.142, No.6, (Dec 2006), pp. 1046-1053, ISSN 0002-9394

Moll, A.C., Imhof, S.M., Bouter, L.M., & Tan, K.E. (1997). Second primary tumors in patients with retinoblastoma. A review of the literature. *Ophthalmic Genet*, Vol.18, No.1, (Mar 1997), pp. 27-34

Moll, A.C., Imhof, S.M., Schouten-Van Meeteren, A.Y., et al. (2001). Second primary tumors in hereditary retinoblastoma: a register-based study, 1945-1997: is there an age effect on radiation-related risk? *Ophthalmology*, Vol.108, No.6, (Jun 2001), pp. 1109-1114, ISSN 0161-6420

Moll, A.C., Imhof, S.M., Schouten-Van Meeteren, A.Y., & Boers, M. (2002). Screening for pineoblastoma in patients with retinoblastoma. *Arch Ophthalmol*, Vol.120, No.12, (Dec 2002), pp. 1774, ISSN 0003-9950

Munier, F.L., Verwey, J., Pica, A., et al. (2008). New developments in external beam radiotherapy for retinoblastoma: from lens to normal tissue-sparing techniques. *Clin Experiment Ophthalmol*, Vol.36, No.1, (Jan-Feb 2008), pp. 78-89, ISSN 1442-6404

Nishimura, S., Sato, T., Ueda, H., & Ueda, K. (2001). Acute myeloblastic leukemia as a second malignancy in a patient with hereditary retinoblastoma. *J Clin Oncol*, Vol.19, No.21, (Nov 2001), pp. 4182-4183, ISSN 0732-183X

Paulino, A.C. Trilateral retinoblastoma: is the location of the intracranial tumor important? *Cancer*, Vol.86, No.1, (Jul 1999), pp. 135-141, ISSN 0008-543X

Pauwels, EK, Bourguignon, M. (2011). Cancer induction caused by radiation due to computed tomography: a critical note. *Acta Radiol*, (Jul 2011), [Epub ahead of print]

Reese, A.B., Hyman, G.A., Merriam, G.R. Jr., et al. (1954). Treatment of retinoblastoma by radiation and triethylenemelamine. *AMA Arch Ophthalmol*, Vol.53, No.4, (Apr 1954), pp. 505-513

Reulen, R.C., Winter, D.L., Frobisher, C., et al; British Childhood Cancer Survivor Study Steering Group. (2010). Long-term cause-specific mortality among survivors of childhood cancer. *JAMA*, Vol.304, No.2, (Jul 2010), pp. 172-179, ISSN 0098-7484

Rieder, H., Lohmann, D., Poensgen, B., et al. (1998). Loss of heterozygosity of the retinoblastoma (RB1) gene in lipomas from a retinoblastoma patient. *J Natl Cancer Inst*, Vol.90, No.4, (Feb 1998), pp. 324-326, ISSN 0027-8874

Rushlow, D., Piovesan, B., Zhang, K., et al. Detection of mosaic RB1 mutations in families with retinoblastoma. *Hum Mutat*, Vol.30, No.5, (May 2009), pp. 842-851, ISSN 1059-7794

Sagerman, R.H., Cassady, J.R., Tretter, P., & Ellsworth, R.M. (1969). Radiation induced neoplasia following external beam therapy for children with retinoblastoma. *Am J Roentgenol Radium Ther Nucl Med*, Vol.105, No.3, (Mar 1969), pp. 529-535, ISSN 0002-9580

Sampieri, K., Mencarelli, M.A., Epistolato, M.C., et al. (2008). Genomic differences between retinoma and retinoblastoma. *Acta Oncol*, Vol. 47, No. 8, (2008), pp. 1483-1492, ISSN 0284-186X

Sanders, B.M., Jay, M., Draper, G.J., & Roberts, E.M. (1989). Non-ocular cancer in relatives of retinoblastoma patients. *Br J Cancer*, Vol.60, No.3, (Sep 1989), pp. 358-365, ISSN 0007-0920

Schlienger, P., Campana, F., Vilcoq, J.R., et al. (2004). Nonocular second primary tumors after retinoblastoma: retrospective study of 111 patients treated by electron beam radiotherapy with or without TEM. *Am J Clin Oncol*, Vol.27, No.4, (Aug 2004), pp. 411-419, ISSN 0277-3732

Sheen, V., Tucker, M.A., Abramson, D.H., et al. (2008). Cancer screening practices of adult survivors of retinoblastoma at risk of second cancers. *Cancer*, Vol.113, No.2, (Jul 2008), pp. 434-441, ISSN 0008-543X

Shields, C.L., Meadows, A.T., Shields, J.A., et al. (2001). Chemoreduction for retinoblastoma may prevent intracranial neuroblastic malignancy (trilateral retinoblastoma). *Arch Ophthalmol*, Vol.119, No.9, (Sep 2001), pp. 1269-1272, ISSN 0003-9950

Sklar, C.A., Mertens, A.C., Mitby, P., et al. (2002). Risk of disease recurrence and second neoplasms in survivors of childhood cancer treated with growth hormone: a report from the Childhood Cancer Survivor Study. *J Clin Endocrinol Metab*, Vol.87, No.7, (Jul 2002), pp. 3136-3141, ISSN 0021-972X

Soh, S.Y., Dimaras, H., Gupta, A., et al. (2011). Adult ovarian retinoblastoma genomic profile distinct from prior childhood eye tumor. *Arch Ophthalmol*, Vol.129, No.8, (Aug 2011), pp. 1101-1104

Strong, L.C., Herson, J., Haas, C., et al. (1984). Cancer mortality in relatives of retinoblastoma patients. *J Natl Cancer Inst*, Vol.73, No.2, (Aug 1984), pp. 303-311, ISBN 0027-8874

Trappey, A., Fernando, A., Gaur, R., et al. (2010). The shady side of sunlight: current understanding of the mechanisms underlying UV-induction of skin cancers. *Front Biosci (Schol Ed)*, Vol.2, (Jan 2010), pp. 11-17

Travis, L.B., Holowaty, E.J., Bergfeldt, K., et al. (1999). Risk of leukemia after platinum-based chemotherapy for ovarian cancer. *N Engl J Med*, Vol.340, No.5, (Feb 1999), pp. 351-357, ISSN 0028-4793

Turaka, K, Shields, CL, Meadows, AT, Leahey, A. (2011). Second malignant neoplasms following chemoreduction with carboplatin, etoposide, and vincristine in 245 patients with intraocular retinoblastoma. *Pediatr Blood Cancer*, (Aug 2011), [Epub ahead of print]

Vázquez, E., Castellote, A., Piqueras, J., et al. (2003). Second malignancies in pediatric patients: imaging findings and differential diagnosis. *Radiographics*, Vol.23, No.5, (Sep-Oct 2003), pp. 1155-1172, ISSN 0271-5333

Weintraub, M., Revel-Vilk, S., Charit, M., et al. (2007). Secondary acute myeloid leukemia after etoposide therapy for retinoblastoma. *J Pediatr Hematol Oncol*, Vol.29, No.9, (Sep 2007), pp. 646-648, ISSN 1077-4114

Wong, F.L., Boice, J.D. Jr., Abramson, D.H., et al. Cancer incidence after retinoblastoma. Radiation dose and sarcoma risk. *JAMA*, Vol. 278, No. 15, (Oct 1997), pp. 1262-1267, ISSN 0098-7484

Woo, K.I., & Harbour, J.W. (2010). Review of 676 second primary tumors in patients with retinoblastoma: association between age at onset and tumor type. *Arch Ophthalmol*, Vol.128, No.7, (Jul 2010), pp. 865-870, ISSN 1538-3601

Yu, C.L., Tucker, M.A., Abramson, D.H., et al. (2009). Cause-specific mortality in long-term survivors of retinoblastoma. *J Natl Cancer Inst*, Vol.101, No.8, (Apr 2009), pp. 581-591, ISSN 0027-8874

Zimmerman, L.E. (1985). Retinoblastoma and retinocytoma. In: *Ophthalmic Pathology: An Atlas and Textbook*. W.H. Spencer, (Ed.), pp. 1292-1351, W.B. Saunders, ISBN 9780721685106, Philadelphia, Pennsylvania

3

Ototoxic Hearing Loss and Retinoblastoma Patients

Shaum P. Bhagat
The University of Memphis
USA

1. Introduction

Chemotherapy is often used in the conservative management of retinoblastoma. Chemotherapy drugs, while ameliorative, can produce long-lasting side effects that potentially can affect survivor quality of life. Carboplatin is a common chemotherapy agent with known ototoxic side effects that is used in the treatment of retinoblastoma (Rodriguez-Galindo et al., 2003). The potential for carboplatin-induced hearing loss is of concern to the medical professional, given that retinoblastoma is often diagnosed in early childhood and children with retinoblastoma have visual impairments. This chapter will outline the mechanisms underlying carboplatin ototoxicity. The extent of knowledge concerning the pathophysiology of carboplatin-induced hearing loss will be explained, and descriptions of the progression of hearing loss on the audiogram will be provided. The types of hearing tests administered to patients receiving carboplatin chemotherapy and monitoring regimens will be reviewed in the chapter. Physiological hearing tests, including the auditory brainstem response (ABR) and otoacoustic emissions (OAE) will be described. Knowledge of these tests will assist the medical professional in understanding if a particular chemotherapy regimen is potentially causing a hearing loss.

The impact of high-frequency hearing loss on the development of speech and language in young children will be discussed, which is of particular relevance in children with an existing visual loss. In the context of this discussion, the academic and social development of children with hearing loss will be addressed. Future directions, including the potential use of otoprotective agents that can be given concurrently with chemotherapy treatment, will be highlighted at the end of the chapter.

2. Pathophysiology of carboplatin-induced hearing loss

Carboplatin (*cis*-diammine [1,1-cyclobutanedicarboxylate]-platinum [II]) is a second-generation platinum compound that initially was reported to have less nephrotoxic and ototoxic side effects than its analog, cisplatin (Bacha et al., 1986). It is a common chemotherapy agent used in the treatment of a wide range of pediatric malignancies. More recently, higher incidences of carboplatin ototoxicity have been reported compared with what was previously described in the literature. The pathophysiology of carboplatin ototoxicity is not completely understood, but evidence from experimental animal models suggests dose-dependent and species-specific effects of carboplatin. Chinchillas are rodents that are commonly used as animal models in experimental studies. In chinchillas, administration of low doses of carboplatin results in the progressive loss of inner hair cells and spiral ganglion neurons from the apex to the base of the cochlea, and outer hair cells are largely unaffected (Takeno et al., 1994; Hofstetter et al., 1997a; Wang et al., 2003; Bauer & Brozoski, 2005). At higher doses of carboplatin, extensive loss of inner hair cells is exhibited across all cochlear turns, and loss of outer hair cells is exhibited most prominently in the basal turn (Hofstetter et al., 1997a; Bauer & Brozoski, 2005). Studies of high-dose carboplatin administration in guinea pigs revealed that primarily outer hair cells were destroyed (Saito et al., 1989), and both outer and inner hair cells were affected in rats (Husain et al., 2001).

3. Methods of hearing assessment in young children

Retinoblastoma is one of the most common intraocular malignancies in young children and it is usually diagnosed before children reach three years of age (Broaddus et al., 2009). Until recently, suspicion of childhood hearing loss was primarily based on behavioral observations by physicians or anecdotes provided by concerned parents. However, reliance on behavioral observations is often confounded by the fact that hearing-impaired infants often seemingly respond to environmental sounds and can babble in a manner similar to normal-hearing infants (Marschark, 1997). These factors often resulted in delays in identifying children with hearing loss. In the past, the typical age of identification of hearing loss in the United States was 11-19 months for children with risk factors for hearing loss and 15-19 months for children with no known risk factors (Mauk et al., 1991; Parving ,1993; Stein, 1995; Harrison & Roush, 1996). In the United Kingdom, the average age of suspicion of hearing loss was 18.8 months and hearing loss was confirmed at an average age of 26 months (Davis et al., 1997). It is crucial that young children with retinoblastoma experiencing vision loss be monitored appropriately while they undergo chemotherapy, as undetected ototoxic hearing loss can impact the development of speech and language.

Hearing is a complex psychological process involving the detection, identification, and comprehension of sound. Assessment of hearing in infants and young children has evolved from reliance primarily on behavioral observations alone to combining behavioral observations with computer-based measurements of auditory physiology. As infants and young children often cannot respond reliably during behavioral hearing assessments, modification of the testing protocol often includes physiological tests of auditory function. While physiological measurements do not test the psychological aspects of hearing directly, they provide information on the status of anatomical structures believed to be crucial for hearing. The major advantage of these physiological tests is that they do not require a behavioral response from the infant, and can be completed rapidly. Most importantly for screening purposes, physiological test results are highly informative in distinguishing between normal-hearing infants and infants with hearing loss. The Joint Committee on Infant Hearing recommended inclusion of ABR and/or OAE tests in screening programs designed to detect hearing loss in infants (Joint Committee on Infant Hearing, 2000). Although these tests are not true tests of hearing, they may provide evidence of a change in cochlear function during the administration of potentially ototoxic medications including carboplatin.

Study	Behavioral Audiometry	ABR	OAE	# of patients studied
Smits et al. (2006)	Yes	Yes	Yes	25
Lambert et al. (2008)	Yes	Yes	No	164
Jehanne et al. (2009)	Yes	No	No	175
Bhagat et al. (2010)	No	No	Yes	10
Pecora Liberman et al. (2011)	Yes	No	Yes	15

Table 1. Recent studies investigating carboplatin ototoxicity in children with retinoblastoma,the monitoring methods used, and the number of patients examined. Yes indicates the test (behavioral audiometry, ABR, OAE) was evaluated in the study and No indicates the test was not evaluated.

3.1 Behavioral assessment of hearing

Assessment of infant hearing involves presentation of sounds through loudspeakers and observing the infant's behavior. If a change in behavior (i.e. the infant is startled) occurs following presentation of a sound, a positive response is noted. The sound level is lowered and the procedure is repeated until no change in behavior is observed. Many infants can respond reliably at sufficiently low levels of sound, and this is suggestive of normal hearing. However, the response of other infants for similar sound levels may be ambiguous. This procedure requires a subjective judgment on whether or not a response has occurred. In addition, many infants cease to respond behaviorally after repeated trials, even though they may be aware of sound in their environment. For these reasons, response detection levels for many infants only provide a gross estimate of hearing sensitivity. However, behavioral observation of infant hearing is useful in corroborating the results of physiological screening tests. For example, if an infant fails an OAE and/or ABR screening, and does not exhibit a behavioral response at sound levels indicative of normal hearing, a hearing loss can be confirmed. In addition, observation of developmental auditory behavior in infants can provide a guideline for comparative purposes. At three months of age, most normal-hearing infants are able to follow the direction a sound is coming from with their eyes. By six months of age, they can turn their heads to determine the source of sounds. If an infant exhibits delays in development of auditory behavior, a hearing loss may be indicated. For older children, hearing may be assessed by visual reinforcement audiometry (VRA) or conditioned play audiometry(CPA). In VRA, a sound is presented through loudspeakers and the child is directed to turn their head in the direction of where the sound came from. Following a correct response, the child is rewarded by seeing an animated toy. This form of reinforcement serves to help the clinician to orient the child to participate in the task and to determine the child's hearing sensitivity. By lowering the sound level until no response is provided by the child, the clinician can obtain an estimate of the hearing threshold on a frequency-by-frequency basis. In CPA, sounds may be presented through loudspeakers or through headphones, and a child is conditioned to drop a block in a bucket (or similar task) every time a sound is heard. Hearing thresholds can be tracked by noting the transitions between sound levels where the child performs or does not perform the task. For both VRA and CPA, the clinician makes a subjective decision to determine whether or not a response occurred, and these methods typically are reserved for children up to 4 years of age. Most older children can participate in a conventional hearing test, whereby they raise their hand or push a button every time they hear a sound, and their responses are noted on a conventional audiogram.

Platinum-compound ototoxicity typically causes hearing loss at audiometric frequencies above 2000 Hz (Macdonald et al., 1994). There are guidelines in place that help to characterize shifts in behavioral hearing thresholds on the audiogram due to the administration of ototoxic medications. Common guidelines in use to characterize ototoxicity in the United States are shown in Table 2. In monitoring ototoxicity, it is vitally important to obtain baseline measurements of hearing before the patient undergoes

Brock	NCI CTCAE	CCG	Chang
Grade 0: < 40 dB at all frequencies		Grade 0: No hearing loss	Grade 0: ≤ 20 dB at 1, 2, and 4 kHz
Grade 1: ≥ 40 dB at 8 kHz only	Grade 1: Threshold shift or loss of 15-25 dB averaged at two contiguous frequencies in one ear	Grade 1: ≥ 40 dB HL loss at 6 kHz and/or 8 kHz	Grade 1a: ≥ 40 dB at any frequency from 6-12 kHz Grade 1b: >20dB and <40 dB at 4 kHz
Grade 2: ≥ 40 dB at 4 kHz and above	Grade 2: Threshold shift or loss >25-90 dB averaged at two contiguous frequencies in one ear	Grade 2: >25 dB HL loss at 3 kHz and/or 4 kHz	Grade 2a: ≥ 40 dB at 4 kHz and above Grade 2b: >20dB and <40 dB at any frequency below 4 kHz
Grade 3: ≥ 40 dB at 2 kHz and above	Grade 3: Hearing loss sufficient to indicate therapeutic intervention, including hearing aids (e.g. > 20 dB bilateral loss in the speech frequencies)	Grade 3: >25 dB HL loss at 2 kHz	Grade 3: ≥ 40 dB at 2 or 3 kHz and above
Grade 4: ≥ 40 dB at 1 kHz and above	Grade 4: Indication for cochlear implant	Grade 4: ≥ 40 dB HL loss at 2 kHz	Grade 4: ≥ 40 dB at 1 kHz and above

Table 2. Common grading scales used in the United States for characterizing ototoxic hearing loss. dB= decibels, dB HL= decibels hearing level, kHz= kiloHertz.

chemotherapy, and then to monitor their hearing at prescribed time points once treatment commences. This allows for comparisons to be made between pre-treatment hearing and peri- or post-treatment hearing in the patient. The Brock grading scale (Brock et al., 1991) assigns a grade based on degree of bilateral hearing loss. The NCI CTCAE (National Cancer Institute Common Terminology Criteria for Adverse Events) uses threshold shifts to assign its grades based on comparisons between baseline and current hearing thresholds. The CCG (Children's Cancer Group) criteria are based on a loss as defined as a change from baseline at any one frequency. The Chang grading scale (Chang & Chinosornvatana, 2010) is the most recent of the grading scales that has been developed.

Clinical studies of carboplatin ototoxicity conducted in children with pediatric cancers other than retinoblastoma have revealed equivocal results. Macdonald et al. (1994) found that 50 % of children in their study had a sensorineural hearing loss in the 4,000-12,000 Hz range following treatment with carboplatin. They found that hearing losses could occur after the first dose of carboplatin, and that hearing losses could progress with subsequent doses. Similarly, Simon et al. (2002) reported that 40% of children treated with high-dose carboplatin developed a hearing impairment and Knight et al. (2005) found that 38% of children treated with carboplatin developed sensorineural hearing loss. In contrast, Stern and Bunin (2002) found that ototoxic complications from carboplatin chemotherapy were rare and mild in severity and other studies have found similar results (Bertolini et al., 2004; Dean et al., 2008). The variability of carboplatin ototoxicity seen across past studies may be related to insufficient control of confounding factors. Factors that may potentiate the severity of carboplatin ototoxicity include prior exposure to cisplatin or other ototoxic medications and high dosage of carboplatin associated with autologous stem cell reinfusion (Knight et al., 2005; Parsons et al., 1998). Another factor that may increase the severity of platinum-compound ototoxicity is patient age, with younger children being more

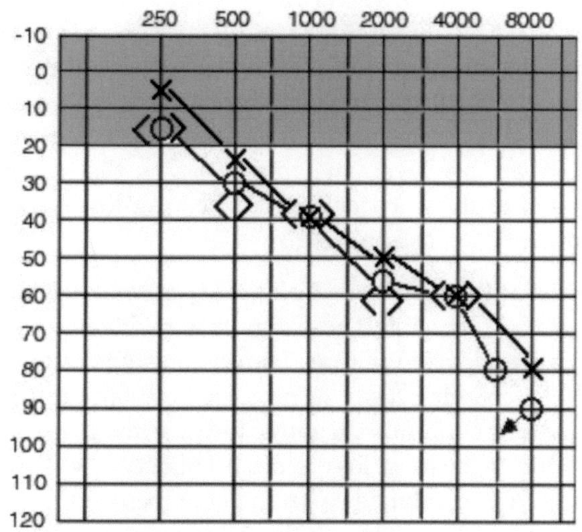

Fig. 1. An audiogram depicting a sensorineural hearing loss in both ears, often seen in ototoxicity. The x-axis is frequency in Hertz and the y-axis is level in decibels. The shaded region represents the normal-hearing range. The hearing loss depicted indicates a greater loss of sensitivity in the high frequencies compared to the low frequencies.

susceptible than older children (Li et al., 2004; Coradini et al., 2007). Studies examining carboplatin ototoxicity in children with retinoblastoma are less prevalent. Smits et al. (2006) studied 25 children diagnosed with retinoblastoma ranging in age from 1-41 months at the start of carboplatin chemotherapy and found no signs of ototoxicity. Lambert et al. (2008) reviewed audiometric data from 116 children (aged 1-87 months) treated for retinoblastoma with a multi-drug regimen including carboplatin. Most of these children were monitored with behavioral audiometry and 48 received ABR evaluations. Only one of the children was suspected of incurring progressive hearing loss due to carboplatin chemotherapy, but this child was diagnosed at less than 1 month of age. Other studies have also indicated a low incidence of carboplatin ototoxicity (4.5-6.6%) in children with retinoblastoma of various ages, although some children were found to have late-onset hearing loss (Jehanne et al., 2009; Pecora Liberman, 2011).

3.2 Auditory brainstem response

Behavioral hearing tests in children less than 12 months old can be unreliable and difficult to interpret. A common alternative method used to monitor auditory function in children receiving platinum-compound chemotherapy is the ABR test. During the ABR test, surface electrodes are attached to locations on the scalp and forehead, and these electrodes record electrical activity generated by the auditory nerve and neural centers in the brain responsive to auditory stimuli. Clicks or brief tones are stimuli presented to an ear while the ABR response is being recorded. The ABR test is a passive test in that the patient does not respond behaviorally to the sounds that are heard. The electrode leads connect to an amplifier box, and the ABR response is filtered and averaged by a computer. The resulting ABR waveform consists of a series of positive and negative voltages displayed on a computer monitor. Peak amplitudes and latencies of the ABR waveform are analyzed and compared to normative data. The lowest level of sound that can evoke a replicable ABR waveform is known as the ABR threshold. Previous research has established that the ABR threshold provides a reliable estimation of infant hearing sensitivity. Children with hearing loss typically have elevated ABR thresholds compared to children with normal hearing. When used as a screening test, a criterion stimulus level is selected and if an ABR waveform is successfully recorded at this level, the infant passes the screening test. If an ABR waveform is not recorded at the criterion level, a hearing loss may be suspected and the infant is referred for further diagnostic testing.

The ABR screening test is a well-established physiological measurement procedure that has been validated through years of clinical research. It is relatively easy to administer and is typically completed in a short period of time. However, as with any screening instrument it is not infallible. The ABR screening test will produce both false positive (incorrectly failing children with normal hearing) and false negative (incorrectly passing children with hearing loss) results. Confirmation of hearing loss is often enhanced when test results from OAE and/or ABR screenings are combined with reliable behavioral observations of infant hearing. In children less than 12 months old, the ABR test may be the only reliable means of examining if auditory function is being compromised by carboplatin, given that younger children receiving platinum compounds may be more susceptible to drug-induced hearing loss as estimated by ABR thresholds (Coupland et al., 1991). Previous research has shown that click-evoked ABR test results can accurately track permanent changes in cochlear function due to administration of ototoxic medications in adults (DeLauretis et al.,1999). However, some studies have questioned the sensitivity of ABR test results in monitoring platinum-compound ototoxicity in children (Weatherly et al., 1991). It is known that carboplatin can cause a substantial amount of damage to inner hair cells and spiral ganglion neurons prior to a change being registered on an electrophysiological assessment, such as the compound action potential (El-Badry & McFadden, 2007). Because the ABR is a far-field potential that relies upon compound activity from an ensemble of neurons, it may not provide the best indication of early change in cochlear function. In addition, if a change is detected on the ABR test, it may reflect a permanent loss of auditory sensitivity.

3.3 Otoacoustic emissions

An alternative method of monitoring platinum-compound ototoxicity is the OAE test. Believed to be linked to the functional status of outer hair cells (Brownell, 1990), OAEs have been effectively used to monitor platinum-compound ototoxicity in children (Dhooge et al., 2006; Knight et al., 2007). OAEs are usually inaudible sounds produced by the healthy inner ear, and these sounds escape into the ear canal and are measured with an ear-canal probe containing a miniature microphone. The probe assembly interfaces with a computer, and a software program analyzes data being recorded by the probe microphone. Typically, OAEs are evoked by stimulating the ear with clicks or tones, and the recorded response is then measured and compared to normative data collected in children with normal hearing. No overt behavioral response from the child is required, and the test can be done while the child is asleep. This physiological test provides information on the functional status of middle and inner ear (outer hair cells) structures. Children with hearing loss have reduced or absent OAEs compared to normal-hearing children. A criterion OAE response is required in order to pass the test, and children who fail are typically referred for further testing to confirm potential hearing loss. The OAE test is a simple screening test to administer and can be completed rapidly, typically within 1-2 minutes per ear. However, a relatively quiet environment is required to complete a valid OAE test, as extraneous noise recorded by the probe microphone can interfere with testing. In addition, the degree of hearing loss cannot be determined by OAE testing alone, as both hard-of-hearing and deaf children typically exhibit absent OAE responses. The information provided by OAE testing is quite useful in determining if a child is a potential candidate for intervention programs.

In children, OAEs were found to be reduced prior to the onset of hearing loss on the audiogram in the conventional frequency range following cisplatin chemotherapy (Knight et al., 2007). DPOAE levels also exhibit high correlations with behavioral hearing thresholds in children suffering hearing loss due to platinum compound ototoxicity (Dhooge et al., 2006). High doses of carboplatin are known to damage outer hair cells and reduce the amplitude of OAEs in animal model (Hofstetter et al., 1997b). Based on these findings, the OAE test potentially is more sensitive at detecting early changes in cochlear function due to carboplatin ototoxicity than is the ABR test. Previous research has not compared the abilities of ABRs and OAEs to register changes in cochlear function throughout the entire course of carboplatin chemotherapy in young children with retinoblastoma. In fact, few studies have examined OAE tests in children with retinoblastoma. Smits et al. (2006) examined OAEs in evaluating children with retinoblastoma receiving carboplatin. They concluded that there were no signs of ototoxicity in the sample of children they examined, although no details concerning what constituted a change in OAE level were provided. Bhagat et al. (2010) found different results in studying 10 children with retinoblastoma receiving carboplatin. They reported that when a criterion change in OAE level was utilized, four of the ten children studied had reductions in OAE level that met the criterion. These findings suggest that OAE tests are useful in identifying the deleterious effects of carboplatin chemotherapy on cochlear function in some children with retinoblastoma.

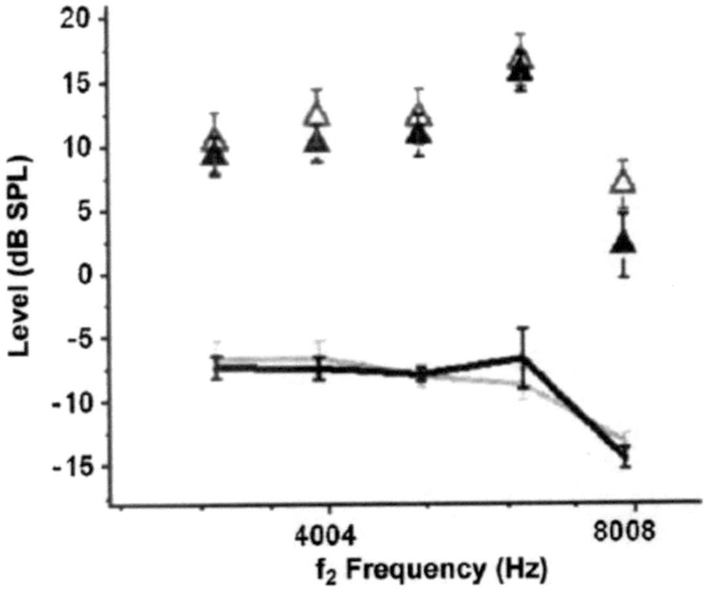

Fig. 2. Mean OAE levels in children with retinoblastoma before (open triangles) and after (filled triangles) carboplatin chemotherapy. Post-therapy OAE levels at the highest test frequency were reduced compared to pre-therapy OAE levels. Reprinted from the International Journal of Pediatric Otorhinolaryngology, Vol. 74/Issue 10, Bhagat, S.P., Bass, J.K., White, S.T., Qaddoumi, I., Wu. J. & Rodriguez-Galindo, C., "Monitoring carboplatin ototoxicity with distortion-product otoacoustic emissions in children with retinoblastoma", pp.1156-1163, 2010, with permission from Elsevier.

4. Impact of hearing loss on academic and social development

The degree of hearing loss associated with carboplatin ototoxicity can vary, but the initial onset of hearing loss typically begins in the high frequencies. High-frequency sensorineural hearing loss can be problematic for the development of speech and language in young children (Stelmachowicz et al., 2004). High frequency speech phonemes contribute to speech intelligibility, and high frequency sensorineural hearing loss reduces the audibility of important speech cues, limits speech understanding in noise, and increases the risk for academic failure (Stelmachowicz et al., 2001; Horwitz et al., 2002; Bess et al., 1998). With more courses or higher dosages of carboplatin, hearing may deteriorate further, and the hearing loss may involve a loss of sensitivity at lower frequencies on the audiogram (Parsons et al., 1998). In rare cases, the use of platinum compounds may result in deafness (Chu et al., 1993).

In most educational settings, the dominant mode of information transfer from teacher to student is oral instruction. Most normal-hearing children have little difficulty understanding oral instruction and have developed a sufficient language base to successfully progress academically. However, children with permanent sensorineural hearing loss are at a disadvantage compared to their normal-hearing peers. Oral instruction may be inaudible to hearing-impaired students, depending upon the degree of hearing loss. In addition, hearing-impaired students often lack language skills that are requisite for achievement in the classroom. While advancements in technology have increased the audibility of classroom instruction for many hearing-impaired students, their expressive and receptive language skills are often below those of children with normal hearing. These language skills form the foundation for word knowledge and verbal reading, which account for 90% of the variability in reading skills found in normal hearing children (Davis, 1972). The lack of an adequate language base in both hard-of-hearing and deaf children impacts their academic performance. Average reading ability for hard-of-hearing high school graduates has been measured at the fifth-grade level, while average reading ability for deaf high school graduates was at the fourth-grade level. Reading ability for both groups was below that of their normal-hearing peers (Allen, 1986). The overall academic performance of hearing-impaired students is negatively influenced by their reading ability (Quigley, 1979).

Once suspected, hearing loss in infants is confirmed through diagnostic tests. The degree of hearing loss can be determined with diagnostic physiological tests such as the ABR combined with behavioral auditory assessments. This information is important, as the type of intervention planned often depends on whether the infant is hard-of-hearing or deaf. Traditional amplification systems, including hearing aids, usually can benefit hard-of-hearing children (Gravel & O'Gara, 2003). When their residual hearing is aided and they are able to hear the acoustic cues of conversational speech, the language acquisition of hard-of-hearing children can be similar to that of normal-hearing children (Moeller, 2000). Factors which influence the language skills of hard-of-hearing children include the age at which their hearing loss was identified, when they received intervention and the amount of parental involvement in the intervention plan (Yoshinaga-Itano et al.,1998; Yoshinaga-Itano & Apuzzo, 1998).

For many deaf children, traditional amplification systems may not be a viable option. These children often do not have enough residual hearing to benefit from hearing aids. Alternative intervention in the form of cochlear implants designed to facilitate development of spoken language, or adoption of manual communication as the child's first language may be more appropriate options. The choice of which communication style to adopt for a deaf child can be a controversial one for many families. This choice can be influenced by the opinions of intervention professionals, who often view deafness as a condition to fix. However, individuals in the Deaf community have argued that deafness is indicative of a cultural difference, and that all deaf children should learn American Sign Language as their primary means of communication (Samson-Fang et al., 2000). The choice of communication style will certainly affect the future educational placement of the deaf child. Deaf children who receive cochlear implants are more likely to be mainstreamed with normal-hearing children in classrooms, while alternative educational placements may be required for children who communicate manually. Regardless of the communication style, evidence indicates that early intervention benefits linguistic outcomes. Children who receive cochlear implants within the age range of 2-6 years perform well on speech reception and production tasks, with better performance seen in children implanted earlier rather than later in life (Brackett & Zara, 1998). Deaf children with early exposure to manual communication developed linguistic skills in a manner similar to normal-hearing children who received early exposure to spoken language (Bandurski & Galkowski, 2004). These findings underscore the importance of early intervention on the development of hearing-impaired children.

Substantial evidence concerning the effects of early identification of hearing loss and early intervention on the language development of hearing-impaired children has been provided by Yoshinaga-Itano and her colleagues. In a series of studies published in peer-reviewed journals, they examined the language skills of children between 13-40 months of age who were identified with hearing loss either before or after the age of six months. The expressive and receptive language development of children enrolled in intervention services before six months of age was significantly better than those of the children identified later in life. Both hard-of-hearing and deaf children benefited from early intervention. Most importantly, the language skills of the early-identified children approached those seen in age-matched normal-hearing children (Yoshinaga-Itano et al., 1998; Yoshinaga-Itano & Apuzzo, 1998). Moeller (2000) extended these results, finding that the benefits of early intervention on language development were maintained in children at five years of age. In addition, personal-social development and self concept are more advanced in children who were identified and enrolled in intervention early in life (Yoshinaga-Itano, 2003).

Another contributing factor to the development of language in hearing-impaired children is the degree of family involvement in the intervention plan (Moeller, 2000). The diagnosis of hearing loss in an infant can be a catastrophic event in the emotional lives of new parents. Parental reaction to this event can contribute significantly to the developmental outcomes for the child (Kurtzer-White & Luterman ,2003). Once they are informed about their child's hearing loss, many parents go through a series of emotions including anger, resentment, and guilt before acceptance of the hearing loss occurs. Recognition of these coping mechanisms by professionals including physicians and educators will enhance parental involvement in the intervention process. There is evidence that well-adjusted families contribute to academic achievement in hearing-impaired children (Feher-Prout, 1996). Educators of the deaf have received training in psychosocial issues of hearing-impaired children and their families, and this expertise can improve the quality of early intervention services.

5. Otoprotection and carboplatin-induced hearing loss

The ability to prevent ototoxicity in patients undergoing carboplatin chemotherapy with pharmaceutical agents is currently being investigated by several teams of researchers. The molecular mechanisms of cell death in the cochlea induced by ototoxic agents are currently being elucidated. Armed with this knowledge, researchers are developing substances that can interrupt the chain of events that lead to hearing loss. These substances are generally known as "otoprotectants". Sodium thiosulfate (STS) is an otoprotectant used to prevent carboplatin ototoxicity that has been evaluated in animal models and in human patients. In guinea pigs, STS was found to reduce the toxicity of carboplatin when it was given up to 8 hours after the ototoxic drug was administered (Neuwelt et al., 1996). Further, the ability of STS to lessen the cochlear toxicity of carboplatin did not interfere with the anti-tumor effectiveness of carboplatin in rats (Muldoon et al., 2000). In a study involving human patients receiving carboplatin, Neuwelt et al. (1998) found that patients given STS 2 hours after carboplatin administration incurred a significantly lower average hearing loss compared with a control group of patients that did not receive STS. The benefits of delayed administration of STS were further revealed when it was shown that when STS is given 4 hours after carboplatin, it reduces ototoxicity rates (Doolittle et al., 2001). The beneficial effects of STS in adults were also seen in a study involving children, where trends indicated that STS provided protection against carboplatin ototoxicity while sparing the anti-tumor activity of the drug (Neuwelt, 2006). Another otoprotectant against carboplatin ototoxicity that has been evaluated in animal models is D-Methionine (D-Met). Lockwood et al. (2000) found that carboplatin-induced cell loss was reduced in chinchillas treated with D-met compared to untreated controls.

In the future, it is conceivable that otoprotectants such as STS or D-Met would be administered during carboplatin chemotherapy in order to reduce the cochlear toxicity of the drug. The use of these pharmaceutical agents to prevent hearing loss would be invaluable in children with retinoblastoma, as these children have existing visual impairments in one or both eyes.

6. Conclusions

Carboplatin is a chemotherapy agent with known ototoxic side effects that is widely used in the conservative management of retinoblastoma. Children with retinoblastoma have visual impairments that may impact their development. There is a risk of incurring additional sensory deficits (loss of hearing) when carboplatin is included in the treatment regimen. Although research to date has indicated a low incidence of carboplatin-induced hearing loss in children with retinoblastoma, additional study of this topic is required before definitive conclusions can be drawn. Factors such as exposure to other ototoxic agents including cisplatin and poor renal function may potentiate carboplatin-induced hearing loss. It is important that medical professionals remain vigilant about monitoring hearing during carboplatin chemotherapy, as conservation of hearing is a priority in children with retinoblastoma. If a change in hearing is noted during the monitoring regimen, it may be possible to alter the dosage of the drug to prevent further deterioration in hearing from occurring. If the carboplatin dose cannot be modified, monitoring hearing status during the treatment regimen can serve as an entry point into intervention programs, including the provision of hearing aids and family counseling. It is also important to note that late-onset hearing loss can occur years after completion of carboplatin chemotherapy. Therefore, long-term hearing assessments may be required in these cases. Recognition of the impact of ototoxic hearing loss on the lives of retinoblastoma survivors will lead to appropriate planning in cases when hearing loss is detected.

7. References

Allen, T. (1986). Patterns of academic achievement among hearing impaired students: 1974 and 1983. In *Deaf Children in America*, A. Schildroth and M. Karchmer, pp.161-206, College Hill Press, ISBN 978-0316483028, Boston, MA, U.S.A.

Bacha, D.M.; Caparros-Sison, B.; Allen, J.A.; Walker, R. & Tan,C.T. (1986). Phase I study of carboplatin (CBDCA) in children with cancer. *Cancer Treatment Reports*, Vol. 70, No. 7 (July 1986), pp. 865-869.

Bandurski, M. & Galkowski, T. (2004). The development of analogical reasoning in deaf children and their parents' communication mode. *Journal of Deaf Studies and Deaf Education,* Vol. 9, No. 2 (Spring 2004), pp. 153-175.

Bauer C.A.& Brozoski T.J. (2005) Cochlear structure and function after round window application of ototoxins. *Hearing Research,* Vol. 201, No.1-2 (March 2005), pp. 121-131.

Bertolini P.; Lasalle M.; Mercier G.; Raquin M.A.; Izzi G.; Corradini N. & Hartmann O. (2004). Platinum compound-related ototoxicity in children: long term follow-up reveals continuous worsening of hearing loss. *Journal of Pediatric Hematology/Oncology,* Vol. 26, No.10 (October 2004), pp.649-655.

Bess, F.H.; Dodd-Murphy, J. & Parker, R.A. (1998). Children with minimal sensorineural hearing loss: prevalence, educational performance and functional status. *Ear and Hearing,* Vol. 1 , No. 5 (October 1998), pp. 339-354.

Bhagat, S.P.; Bass, J.K.; White, S.T.; Qaddoumi, I.; Wilson, M.W.; Wu, J. & Rodriguez-Galindo, C. (2010). Monitoring carboplatin ototoxicity with distortion-product otoacoustic emissions in children with retinoblastoma. *International Journal of Pediatric Otorhinolaryngology,* Vol. 74, No. 10 (October 2010), pp. 1156-1163.

Brackett, D. & Zara, C. (1998). Communication outcomes related to early implantation. *Am erican Journal of Otology,* Volume 19, No. 4 (July 1998), pp. 453-460.

Broaddus E.; Topham A. & Singh A.D. (2009) Incidence of retinoblastoma in the USA: 1975-2004. *British Journal of Ophthalmology,* Vol.93, No. 1 (January 2009), pp. 21-23.

Brock, P.R.; Bellman, S.C.; Yeomans, E.C.; Pinkerton, C.R. & Pritchard, J. (1991). Cisplatin ototoxicity in children: a practical grading system. *Medical and Pediatric Oncology,* Vol. 19, No. 4, pp.295-300.

Brownell, W.E. (1990). Outer hair cell electromotility and otoacoustic emissions. *Ear and Hearing,* Vol.11, No. 2 (April 1990), pp. 82-92.

Chang, K.W. & Chinosornvatana, N. (2010). Practical grading system for evaluating cisplatin ototoxicity in children. *Journal of Clinical Oncology,* Vol. 28, No. 10 (March 2010), pp.1788-1795.

Chu, G.; Mantin, R.; Shen, Y.M.; Baskett, G. & Sussman, H. (1993). Massive cisplatin overdose by accidental substitution for carboplatin. Toxicity and management. *Cancer,* Vol. 72, No. 12 (December 1993) pp.3707-3714.

Coradini, P.P.; Cigana L.; Selistre S.G.; Rosito, L.S. & Brunetto, AL. (2007) Ototoxicity from cisplatin therapy in childhood cancer. *Journal of Pediatric Hematology/Oncology,* Vol. 29, No. 6 (June 2007), pp. 355-360.

Coupland, S.G; Ponton, C.W.; Eggermont, J.J.; Bowen, T.J. & Grant, R.M. (1991). Assessment of cisplatin-induced ototoxicity using derived-band ABRs. *International Journal of Pediatric Otorhinolaryngology,* Vol. 22, No. 3 (October 1991), pp. 237-248.

Davis, F. (1972). Psychometric research on comprehension in reading. *Reading Research Quarterly,* Vol. 7, pp. 628-678.

Davis, A.; Bamford, J.; Wilson, I.; Ramkalawan, T.; Forshaw, M. & Wright, S. (1997). A critical review of the role of neonatal hearing screening in the detection of congenital hearing impairment. *Heath Technology Assessment,* Vol. 1, No. 10, pp. 1-176.

Dean J.B.; Hayashi S.S.; Albert C.M.; King A.A.; Karson R. & Hayashi R.J. (2008). Hearing loss in pediatric oncology patients receiving carboplatin-containing regimens. *Journal of Pediatric Hematology/ Oncology* Vol. 30, No. 2 (February 2008), pp.130-134.

DeLauretis, A., De Capua, B., Barbieri, M.T., Bellussi, L., & Passali, D. (1999). ABR evaluation of ototoxicity in cancer patients receiving cisplatin or carboplatin. *Scandinavian Audiology*, Vol. 28, No. 3, pp. 139-143.

Dhooge, I., Dhooge, C., Geukens, S., De Clerck, B., De Vel, E., & Vinck, B.M. (2006). Distortion product otoacoustic emissions: an objective technique for the screening of hearing loss in children treated with platin derivatives. *International Journal of Audiology*, Vol. 45, No. 6 (June 2006), pp. 337-343.

Doolittle, N.D.; Muldoon, L.L.; Brummett, R.E.; Tyson, R.M.; Lacy, C.; Bubalo, J.S.; Kraemer, D.F.; Heinrich, M.C.; Henry, J.A. & Neuwelt, E.A.(2001). Delayed sodium thiosulfate as an otoprotectant against carboplatin-induced hearing loss in patients with malignant brain tumors. *Clinical Cancer Research*, Vol. 7, No. 3 (March 2001), pp. 493-500.

El-Badry, M.M. & McFadden, S.L. (2007). Electrophysiological correlates of progressive sensorineural pathology in carboplatin-treated chinchillas. *Brain Research* , Vol. 1134, No. 1 (January 2007), pp.122-130.

Feher-Prout, T. (1996). Stress and coping in families with deaf children. *Journal of Deaf Studies and Deaf Education*, Vol. 1, pp. 155-165.

Gravel, J. & O'Gara, J. (2003). Communication options for children with hearing loss. Vol. 9, pp. 243-251.

Harrison, M. & Roush, J. (1996). Age of suspicion, identification and intervention for infants and young children with hearing loss. *Ear and Hearing*, Vol.17 ,No. 1(February 1996), pp. 55-62.

Hofstetter, P.; Ding, D. & Salvi, R. (1997a). Magnitude and pattern of inner and outer hair cell loss in chinchilla as a function of carboplatin dose. *Audiology*, Vol. 36, No.6 (November-December 1997), pp. 301-311.

Hofstetter, P., Ding, D., Powers, N., & Salvi, R. (1997b). Quantitative relationship of carboplatin dose to magnitude of inner and outer hair cell loss and the reduction of distortion product otoacoustic emission amplitude in chinchillas. *Hearing Research*, Vol.112, No. 1-2 (October 1997), pp.199-215.

Horwitz, A.R., Dubno, J.R., & Ahlstrom, J.B. (2002). Recognition of low-pass-filtered consonants in noise with normal and impaired high frequency hearing. *The Journal of the Acoustical Society of America*, Vol. 111 ,No. 1 (January 2002), pp. 409-416.

Husain, K.; Whitworth, C.; Somari, S.M. & Rybak, L.P. (2001). Carboplatin-induced oxidative stress in rat cochlea. *Hearing Research*, Vol.159, No. 1-2 (September 2001), pp.14-22.

Jehanne, M.; Lumbroso-Le Rouic, L.; Savignoni, A.; Aerts, I.; Mercier, G.; Bours, D.; Desjardins, L & Doz, F. (2009). Analysis of ototoxicity in young children receiving carboplatin in the context of conservative management of unilateral or bilateral retinoblastoma. *Pediatric Blood and Cancer*, Vol. 52, No. 5 (May 2009), pp. 637-643.

Joint Committee on Infant Hearing (2000). Year 2000 position statement: principles and guidelines for early hearing detection and intervention programs. *American Journal of Audiology* , Vol.9, No.1 (June 2000), pp. 9-29.

Knight, K.R.; Kraemer, D.F. & Neuwelt, E.A. (2005). Ototoxicity in children receiving platinum chemotherapy: underestimating a commonly occurring toxicity that may influence academic and social development. *Journal of Clinical Oncology*, Vol.23, No. 34 (December 2005), pp.8588-8596.

Knight, K.R.; Kraemer, D.F.; Winter, C. & Neuwelt, E.A. (2007). Early changes in auditory function as a result of platinum chemotherapy: use of extended high-frequency audiometry and evoked distortion product otoacoustic emissions. *Journal of Clinical Oncology*, Vol.25, No. 10 (April 2007), pp. 1190-1195.

Kurtzer-White, E. & Luterman, D. (2003). Families and children with hearing loss: grief and coping. *Mental Retardation and Developmental Disabilities Research Review,* Vol. 9, pp. 232-235.

Lambert, M.P.; Shields, C & Meadows, A.T. (2008). A retrospective review of hearing in children with retinoblastoma treated with carboplatin-based chemotherapy. *Pediatric Blood and Cancer,* Vol. 50, No. 2 (February 2008), pp.223-236.

Li, Y.; Womer, R.B. & Silber, J.H. (2004). Predicting cisplatin ototoxicity in children: the influence of age and the cumulative dose. *European Journal of Cancer,* Vol 40, No. 16 (November 2004), pp. 2445-2551.

Lockwood, D.S.; Ding, D.L.; Wang, J. & Salvi, R.J. (2000). D-Methionine attenuates inner hair cell loss in carboplatin-treated chinchillas. *Audiology and Neuro-otology,* Vol. 5, No. 5 (September-October 2000), pp.263-266.

Macdonald, M.R.; Harrison, R.V.; Wake, M.; Bliss, B. & Macdonald, R.E. (1994). Ototoxicity of carboplatin: comparing animal and clinical models at the Hospital for Sick Children. *Journal of Otolaryngology,* Vol. 23, No. 3 (June 1994), pp.151-159.

Marschark, M.(1997). *Psychological Development of Deaf Children,* Oxford Univ. Press, ISBN 978-0195115758, Oxford, England.

Mauk, G.; White, K.; Mortensen, L. & Behrens, T. (1991). The effectiveness of screening programs based on high-risk characteristics in early identification of hearing loss. *Ear and Hearing,* Vol. 12 , No. 5 (October 1991), pp. 312-319.

Moeller, M. (2000). Early intervention and language development in children who are deaf and hard of hearing. *Pediatrics,* Vol.106, No. 3 (September 2000), pp. E43.

Muldoon, L.L.; Pagel, M.A.; Kroll, R.A.; Brummett, R.E.; Doolittle, N.D.; Zuhowski, E.G.; Egorin, M.J.; Neuwelt, E.A. (2000). Delayed administration of sodium thiosulfate in animal models reduces platinum ototoxicity without reduction of antitumor activity. *Clinical Cancer Research,* Vol. 6, No. 1 (January 2000), pp. 309-315.

Neuwelt, E.A.; Brummett, R.E.; Remsen. L.G.; Kroll, R.A.; Pagel, M.A.; McCormick, C.I.; Guitjens, S. & Muldoon, L.L. (1996). In vitro and animal studies of sodium thiosulfate as a potential chemoprotectant against carboplatin-induced ototoxicity. *Cancer Research,* Vol. 56, No. 4 (February 1996), pp. 706-709.

Neuwelt, E.A.; Brummett, R.E.; Doolittle, N.D.; Muldoon, L.L.; Kroll, R.A.; Pagel, M.A.; Dojan, R.; Church, V.; Remsen, L.G.& Bubalo, J.S. (1998), First evidence of otoprotection against carboplatin–induced hearing loss with a two-compartment system in patients with central nervous system malignancy using sodium thiosulfate. *The Journal of Pharmacology and Experimental Therapeutics,* Vol. 286, No. 1 (July 1998), pp. 77-84.

Neuwelt, E.A.; Gilmer-Knight, K.; Lacy, C.; Nicholson, H.S.; Kraemer, D.F.; Doolittle, N.D.; Hornig, G.W. & Muldon, L.L. (2006). *Pediatric Blood and Cancer,* Vol. 47, No.2 (August 2006), p.174-182.

Parsons, S.K.; Neault, M.W.; Lehmann, L.E.; Brennan, L.L;, Eickhoff, C.E.; Kretschmar, C.S. & Diller, L.R. (1998). Severe ototoxicity following carboplatin-containing conditioning regimen for autologous marrow transplantation for neuroblastoma. *Bone Marrow Transplantation*, Vol.22, No. 7 (October 1998), pp. 669-674.

Parving, A. (1993). Congenital hearing disability: epidemiology and identification- a comparison between two health authority districts. *International Journal of Pediatric Otorhinolaryngology*, Vol. 27, No. 1 (May 1993), pp.29-46.

Pecora Liberman, P.H.; Schultz, C.; Schmidt Goffi-Gomez, M.V.; Antonelli, C.B.; Motoro Chojniak, M.& Eduardo Novaes, P. (2011). Evaluation of ototoxicity in children treated for retinoblastoma :preliminary results of a systematic audiological evaluation. *Clinical and Translational Oncology*, Vol. 13, No. 5 (May 2011), pp. 348-352.

Quigley, S. (1979). Environment and communication in the language development of deaf children. In *Hearing and Hearing Impairment*, L. Bradford and W. Hardy ,pp. 287-298, Grune and Stratton, ISBN 978-0808911456, New York, N.Y., U.S.A.

Rodriguez-Galindo, C.; Wilson, M.W.; Haik, B.G.; Merchant, T.E.; Billups, C.A.; Shah, N.; Cain, A.; Langston, J.; Lipson, M.; Kun, L.E. & Pratt, C.B. (2003). Treatment of intraocular retinoblastoma with vincristine and carboplatin. *Journal of Clinical Oncology*, Vol.21, No.10 (May 2003), pp.2019-2025.

Saito, T.; Saito, H; Saito, K.; Wakui, S. Manabe, Y. & Tsuda, G. (1989). Ototoxicity of carboplatin in guinea pigs. *Auris, Nasus, Larynx* , Vol.16, No. 1, pp. 13-21.

Samson-Fang, L.; Simons-McCandless, M. & Shelton, C. (2000). Controversies in the field of hearing impairment: early identification, educational methods and cochlear implants. *Infants and Young Children*, Vol.12, pp. 77-88.

Simon, T.; Hero, B.; Dupuis, W.; Selle, B. & Berthold, F. (2002). The incidence of hearing impairment after successful treatment of neuroblastoma. *Klinische Padiatrie*, Vol. 214, No. 4 (July-August 2002), pp. 149-152.

Smits, C.; Swen, S.J.; Goverts, S.T.; Moll, A.C.; Imhof, S.K. & Schouten-van Meeteren, A. (2006). Assessment of hearing in very young children receiving carboplatin for retinoblastoma. *European Journal of Cancer*, Vol.42, No. 4 (March 2006), pp. 492-500.

Stein, L. (1995). On the real age of identification of congenital hearing loss. *Audiology Today*, Vol. 7, pp.10-11.

Stelmachowicz, P.G.; Pittman, A.L.; Hoover, B.M. & Lewis, D.E. (2001). Effect of stimulus bandwidth on the perception of /s/ in normal and hearing-impaired children and adults. *The Journal of the Acoustical Society of America*, Vol. 110, No. 4 (October 2001), pp. 2183-2190.

Stelmachowicz, P.G.; Pittman, A.L.; Hoover, B.M.; Lewis, D.E. & Moeller, M.P. (2004). The importance of high-frequency audibility in the speech and language development of children with hearing loss. *Archives of Otolaryngology-Head and Neck Surgery*, Vol. 130, No. 5 (May 2004), pp. 556-562.

Stern, J.W. & Bunin, N. (2003). Prospective study of carboplatin-based chemotherapy for pediatric germ cell tumors. *Medical and Pediatric Oncology*, Vol. 39, No. 3 (September 2002), pp.163-167.

Takeno, S.; Harrison, R.V.; Ibrahim, D.; Wake, M. & Mount, R.J. (1994). Cochlear function after selective inner hair cell degeneration induced by carboplatin. *Hearing Research*, Vol. 75, No.1-2 (May 1994) pp.93-102.

Wang, J.; Ding, D, & Salvi, R.J. (2003). Carboplatin-induced early cochlear lesion in chinchillas. *Hearing Research*, Vol. 181, No.1-2 (July 2003), p.65-72.

Weatherly, R.A.; Owens, J.J.; Caitlin, F.I. & Mahoney, D.H. (1991). Cis-platin ototoxicity in children. *Laryngoscope* , Vol. 101, No. 9 (September 1991), pp.917-924.

Yoshinaga-Itano, C. (2003). From screening to early identification and intervention: discovering predictors to successful outcomes for children with significant hearing loss. *Journal of Deaf Studies and Deaf Education,* Vol. 8, pp. 11-30.

Yoshinaga-Itano C. & Apuzzo, M. (1998). Identification of hearing loss after age 18 months is not early enough. *American Annals of the Deaf* , Vol.143, pp. 380-387.

Yoshinaga-Itano, C.; Sedey, A.L.; Coulter, D.K. & Mehl, AL. (1998). Language of early- and later-identified children with hearing loss. *Pediatrics,* Vol. 102, No. 5 (November 1998), pp. 1161-1171.

4

Retinoblastoma – Genetic Counseling and Molecular Diagnosis

Claude Houdayer[1,4], Marion Gauthier-Villars[1], Laurent Castéra[1], Laurence Desjardins[2], François Doz[3,4] and Dominique Stoppa-Lyonnet[1,4,5]
[1]Genetics Department, Institut Curie, Paris
[2]Ophtalmology Department, Institut Curie, Paris
[3]Pediatrics Department, Institut Curie, Paris
[4]Université Paris Descartes, Paris
[5]INSERM U830, Pathologie Moléculaire des Cancers, Institut Curie, Paris
France

1. Introduction

Retinoblastoma is a malignant embryonal tumour of childhood arising at the expense of retinal cones. It has an incidence of 1 per 15,000 to 20,000 births. In 90% of cases, it is diagnosed before the age of 3 years. The possibility of conservative management depends on early diagnosis (Moll et al., 1996). However, although treatment strategies have advanced considerably, the visual prognosis is still a major source of concern, especially central vision when the tumour is situated at or close to the macula. In two-thirds of cases, the lesion is unilateral and the median age of diagnosis is 2 years. In the other third, the lesion is bilateral and the disease is diagnosed earlier, possibly even during the neonatal period, with a median age of diagnosis of 1 year. Most cases of unilateral and bilateral retinoblastoma are sporadic, with no family history. However, 10 to 15% of all cases of retinoblastoma present a family history. The distribution of cases within the family is compatible with the existence of a tumour susceptibility gene transmitted according to an autosomal dominant mode with high penetrance. In this case, the lesion is usually bilateral and diagnosed at an early age.

1.1 Diagnosis

The most frequent presenting signs are leukocoria (white pupillary reflex) and strabismus. Retinoblastoma may also be discovered on routine ocular fundus examination performed in a child from a high-risk family.

The diagnosis is essentially based on the ocular fundus examination under general anaesthesia, completed by ultrasound and CT. Tumour growth may be endophytic with invasion of the vitreous cavity or, more rarely, exophytic with retinal detachment. A precise description of the lesions based on fundoscopy findings allows the lesion to be classified according to the 5 stages of the Reese-Ellsworth classification, associated with an increasingly severe prognosis. Ultrasound and orbital CT demonstrate tumour calcifications highly suggestive of retinoblastoma and CT contributes to staging in advanced forms. In the case of enucleation, the diagnosis and staging are confirmed by histological criteria.

Conservative treatment must be attempted whenever possible: chemotherapy, radiotherapy, photocoagulation, and cryotherapy. Very advanced forms unsuitable for conservative treatment will require enucleation. This treatment is still unfortunately often required for sporadic retinoblastomas whose diagnosis is made late.

1.2 Predisposition to retinoblastoma

In 1971, Knudson proposed a model designed to explain why most familial retinoblastomas were bilateral and occurred at an early age and, inversely, why unilateral cases were usually isolated and diagnosed later (Knudson, 1971). He proposed the hypothesis that two mutations of key genes in the control of cell division occurring in a retinal neuroectodermal cell were necessary, but possibly not sufficient, for development of retinoblastoma. In bilateral forms, the first mutation is a germline mutation, present in all cells of the body and especially in all retinal neuroectodermal embryonal cells, while the second mutation is somatic, acquired during foetal life or the first months of neonatal life. Although the probability of two somatic mutations in two key genes in the same retinal cell is extremely low, development of a single mutation is not a rare event and induces development of a retinoblastoma when another mutation is already present. This explains why children with a germline mutation have a high risk of developing not just one, but two or more tumours. Comings completed Knudson's hypothesis in 1973 by postulating that the two mutations necessary for the development of retinoblastoma corresponded to inactivation of the two alleles of the same gene, that had not yet been identified at that time (Comings, 1973). The hypothesis of the existence of tumour suppressor genes, already suspected, became very likely.

In familial cases, the germline mutation is transmitted by one of the parents. In sporadic, bilateral and sometimes multifocal unilateral cases, the germline mutation usually corresponds to a *de novo* mutation arising in the gametes of one of the two parents (pre-zygotic) or at an early stage after fertilization (post-zygotic). Pre-zygotic *de novo* mutations are associated with advanced paternal age. In some cases, the apparently sporadic nature of retinoblastoma is related to incomplete penetrance in one carrier parent. As the risk of tumour is high, but incomplete, a parent with a germline mutation may fail to develop retinoblastoma during childhood or may have developed a spontaneously regressive retinoblastoma, which may leave a retinal scar or retinoma. It is therefore very important to perform an ocular fundus examination in each parent looking for retinoma, which would reveal a previously unknown family history that would consequently modify genetic counseling. This point is discussed in more detail in the "Notes" section of the chapter on "Genetic counseling".

Most unilateral cases are due to two mutations occurring only at the somatic level. However, it is estimated that almost 10% of patients with unilateral retinoblastoma have a germline mutation.

A risk of cancer different of retinoblastoma exists within retinoblastoma predisposition. Rare patients develop pineal region tumour but is considered like an ectopic intracranial retinoblastoma and so-called trilateral retinoblastoma. An increased risk of second cancers for *RB1* mutation carriers, after retinoblastoma, is well documented. In childhood and early adulthood, these patients have a high incidence of osteosarcomas and soft tissue sarcomas. The incidence of these cancers can often be attributed to external beam radiation therapy, but many cases have been reported occurring outside of the field of radiation treatment and even for patients who received no radiation. A cumulative rate of second cancers is reported 18 years after the diagnosis of genetic retinoblastoma at 8.4% (and 6% for osteosarcomas alone) (Draper et al., 1986). Otherwise, *RB1* mutation carriers have also a high lifetime risk of developing a late onset epithelial cancer (lung, bladder, breast) and melanoma. In a historic series of 144 survivors of hereditary retinoblastomas, the cumulative cancer incidence to 85 years of age has been estimated to be 68.8% (CI= 48.0% to 87.4%) (Fletcher et al., 2004).

1.3 The *RB1* gene

The identification, in 1963, of germline deletions of chromosome 13 (then considered to be a group D chromosome) in rare patients with bilateral retinoblastoma and presenting mental retardation and a dysmorphic syndrome suggested that the retinoblastoma susceptibility gene was localized in this chromosomal region (Baud et al., 1999, Lele et al., 1963). Comparative analysis of highly polymorphic germline and tumour genetic markers localized in 13q14 subsequently demonstrated loss of heterozygosity in about 65% of tumours. In other words, in more than one half of tumours, the susceptibility gene is altered in somatic cells by complete loss of the chromosomal region in which it is localized. It has also been demonstrated that, in familial forms of retinoblastoma, the remaining allele in the tumour was always the allele common to all affected members of the family, i.e. the allele carrying the predisposition to retinoblastoma. Analysis of a large number of retinoblastomas identified the smallest common region of deletion in 13q14, which allowed research to be focussed on this region. In 1986, identification of a gene localized in the region of interest and constituting a site of inactivating germline mutations in children with bilateral retinoblastoma confirmed that this gene corresponded to the retinoblastoma susceptibility gene; it was called *RB1*(Friend et al., 1986). Identification of *RB1* confirmed the complementary hypotheses of Knudson and Comings, opened the way to cancer susceptibility gene testing and allowed definition of the risk of retinoblastoma within particular families.

The *RB1* gene codes for a 110 kD nuclear protein with an ubiquitous expression, which, together with proteins p107 and p130, belongs to the pocket protein family. These proteins share in common a domain corresponding to a highly conserved region, the pocket domain, which allows sequestration of transcription factors, such as those of the E2F family. During the G1/S transition of the cell cycle, the pRB protein binds to E2F factors and suppresses their activity, consequently blocking progression to S phase. Inversely, phosphorylation of pRB releases E2F factors, allowing completion of the cell cycle. The pRB protein is involved not only in regulation of the cell cycle, but also in control of termination of cellular differentiation and in exit of the cell from the cell cycle during development. It appears to interact with more than 100 different proteins (Zhu, 2005, Classon&Harlow, 2002, Chau&Wang, 2003, Bremner et al., 2004). It is probably this role in differentiation which explains the spatiotemporal specificity of the tumour risk associated with *RB1* gene mutations and consequently damage to retinal neuroectodermal cells during early childhood.

2. Genetic counseling protocols

2.1 Overview

Whenever unilateral or bilateral retinoblastoma is diagnosed in a child, it is important to consider the possibility of a genetic predisposition and therefore the risk of development of the disease in young children related to the patient.

Analysis of the family history and the tumour history of a patient treated for retinoblastoma is essential to evaluate the possibility of a genetic predisposition and the risk of development of the disease in other members of the child's family and to guide the ophthalmological surveillance of family members (siblings, cousins or offspring). It is therefore possible to calculate the probability of relatives of a child with retinoblastoma to present a genetic predisposition to this disease. These calculations are based on the following elements: (1) 100% of patients with bilateral retinoblastoma and 10% of patients with unilateral retinoblastoma are considered to present a genetic predisposition, (2) the mode of transmission is dominant; a carrier parent therefore has once chance in two of transmitting the susceptibility gene to each child, (3) the penetrance is 90% at birth, which means that an adult who did not develop retinoblastoma in childhood has a tenfold lower probability of being a carrier compared to the probability at birth (Figure 1).

Based on comparative analysis of the various approaches to ophthalmological surveillance in different countries and our multidisciplinary experience at Institut Curie, we can propose guidelines for the surveillance of relatives of patients followed for retinoblastoma (Figure 1) (Abramson et al., 1998, Moll et al., 2000, Musarella&Gallie, 1987). The modalities of this surveillance depend on the probability of predisposition of the child to be followed, which depends on the child's age and degree of kinship with the affected child, and on the age distribution at diagnosis in predisposed children followed since birth. In a series of 50 predisposed children followed since birth, the diagnosis of retinoblastoma was established before the age of 6 months in 80% of cases, before the age of 18 months in 92% of cases and at the age of 4 years in one case. Finally, even for the lowest levels of risk for which ophthalmological surveillance is recommended, ocular fundus examination must be performed at least every 3 months until the age of 24 months in order to ensure effective prevention. These surveillance guidelines are very rigorous: ocular fundus examination at the first month of life, or even the first week, in a specialized unit, with frequent follow-up examinations requiring general anaesthesia from the second or third examination. For example, in the case of a 50% risk of being a carrier (a child born to a patient with bilateral retinoblastoma), surveillance starts at the first week of life, and then once a month until the age of 18 months (Figure 1).

These guidelines must be maintained in the absence of genetic testing or while waiting for the results, as genetic testing in all patients with unilateral or bilateral retinoblastoma, followed by testing of the relatives, can eliminate the need for surveillance of a certain number of children, depending on the results.

2.2 Counseling

Molecular genetic studies of the *RB1* gene can now be proposed to all patients with familial or sporadic unilateral or bilateral retinoblastoma. Genetic testing must be performed in the

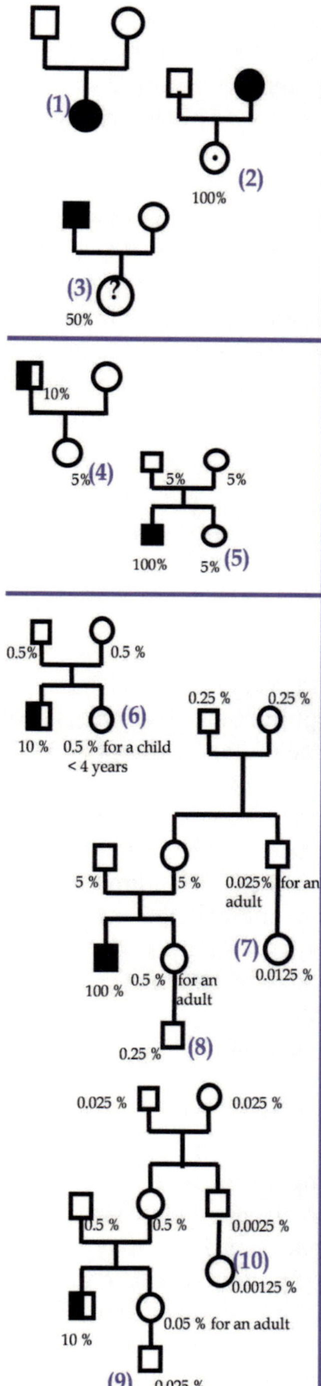

(1)Patient with unilateral or bilateral retinoblastoma

Risk of retinoblastoma between 50% and 100%

(2) Unaffected child with a *RBI* gene mutation

(3) Offspring of a patient presumed to have a *RBI* gene mutation (patient with bilateral or multifocal unilateral or familial retinoblastoma) with no identified *RBI* gene mutation

First week of life (unaffected infant)
Every month until the age of 18 months
Gradually prolong intervals to every 3 months until the age of 4 years
Every 4 to 6 months until the age of 20
Annually for life

Risk of retinoblastoma of 5% (1/20)

(4) Offspring of a patient with unilateral, unifocal, non-familial retinoblastoma

(5) Siblings of a patient with bilateral or multifocal unilateral, non-familial retinoblastoma

First month of life
Every 2 months until the age of 4 years
Every 6 months until the age of 4 years
Annually until the age of 20

Risk of retinoblastoma of about 0.5% (1/200) to 0.0125% (1/8,000)

(6) Siblings of a patient with unilateral,unifocal, non-familial retinoblastoma,
(7) Second cousins of a patient with non-familial bilateral retinoblastoma
(8) Nephews and nieces of a patient with non-familial bilateral retinoblastoma
(9) Nephews and nieces of a patient with non-familial unilateral retinoblastoma

First month of life
Every 3 months until the age of 2 years
Every 6 months until the age of 4 years

Risk of retinoblastoma of about 0.005% (1/20,000)
(~ risk in the general population)

(10) Second cousins of a patient with non-familial unilateral retinoblastoma

No follow-up required

Risk calculations take into account the fact that: (1) 100% of patients with bilateral retinoblastoma and 10% of patients with unilateral retinoblastoma are carriers, (2) dominant transmission, (3) 90% penetrance at birth; the corollary is that an adult who did not develop retinoblastoma during childhood has a tenfold lower probability of being a carrier compared to the probability at birth.

■ bilateral retinoblastoma

◧ unilateral retinoblastoma

Fig. 1. Ophthalmological surveillance guidelines

context of a genetics consultation in collaboration with the ophthalmology, paediatric oncology and radiotherapy teams managing the child. During this consultation, the patient's pedigree is built looking for other tumour cases in the family and especially other retinoblastoma cases. Patient or parents of young patients are informed about retinoblastoma predisposition. Ocular fundus examination of parents is required to search for retinoma which would reveal a previously unknown family history. Follow up of young patient's relatives by ocular fundus is recommended. Blood sampling for *RB1* molecular analysis is proposed to search for germline mutation. Finally, an informed consent has to be signed by the patients or their legal guardians if *RB1* screening is accepted. Following *RB1* screening, results are delivered during another genetic consultation. The printed test results are given to the parents and are also kept by the genetics department for at least thirty years, so that they can be consulted by the child during early adulthood. Today, a first-line screening for the two inactivating somatic mutations in the tumor DNA (when available) is performed and represents an attractive alternative: identification of these mutations only in the tumour and not in the leukocytes of the patient eliminates the risk of recurrence in siblings and cousins (see below).

The assessment usually starts with molecular genetic testing but cytogenetic analysis is performed as first-line procedure in the case of associated mental retardation or characteristic dysmorphic syndrome.

2.3 Clinical management/surveillance (Figure 2)

When a mutation has been demonstrated in an affected child, genetic testing based on screening for this mutation, is recommended for the siblings. Ophthalmological surveillance can be stopped in a relative when genetic testing fails to reveal the mutation identified in the family. Genetic testing is also proposed to the parents. If one of the two parents carries the mutation, antenatal diagnosis may be proposed for a subsequent pregnancy. If the parents do not carry the mutation, their respective families can be reassured, eliminating the need for ophthalmological surveillance of the patient's cousins. In contrast, it is impossible to assess the level of representation of the mutation identified in the affected child in the gametes of the parent in which a *de novo* mutation has occurred (quantification of the germline mosaic), or, in other words, it is impossible to eliminate the risk of recurrence in the siblings of the affected child. In this case, for each new birth in the immediate family, a genetic test must be proposed during the neonatal period. Antenatal diagnosis can be proposed case by case.

When no *RB1* gene mutation is demonstrated in the affected child:

1. In the case of bilateral retinoblastoma, genetic screening techniques have certain limitations and may fail to demonstrate a mutation, in which case surveillance of the patient's relatives must be continued (Figure 1). Somatic mosaics may also be observed, as an alteration of the *RB1* gene can occur in the patient during embryonic development and may not be present in leukocyte DNA. If the mutation is present in the germline, this patient may transmit the mutation to his/her offspring. It is currently proposed to repeat *RB1* gene testing at the birth of each child of a patient with a history of bilateral retinoblastoma in childhood in whom molecular *RB1* gene testing was negative.

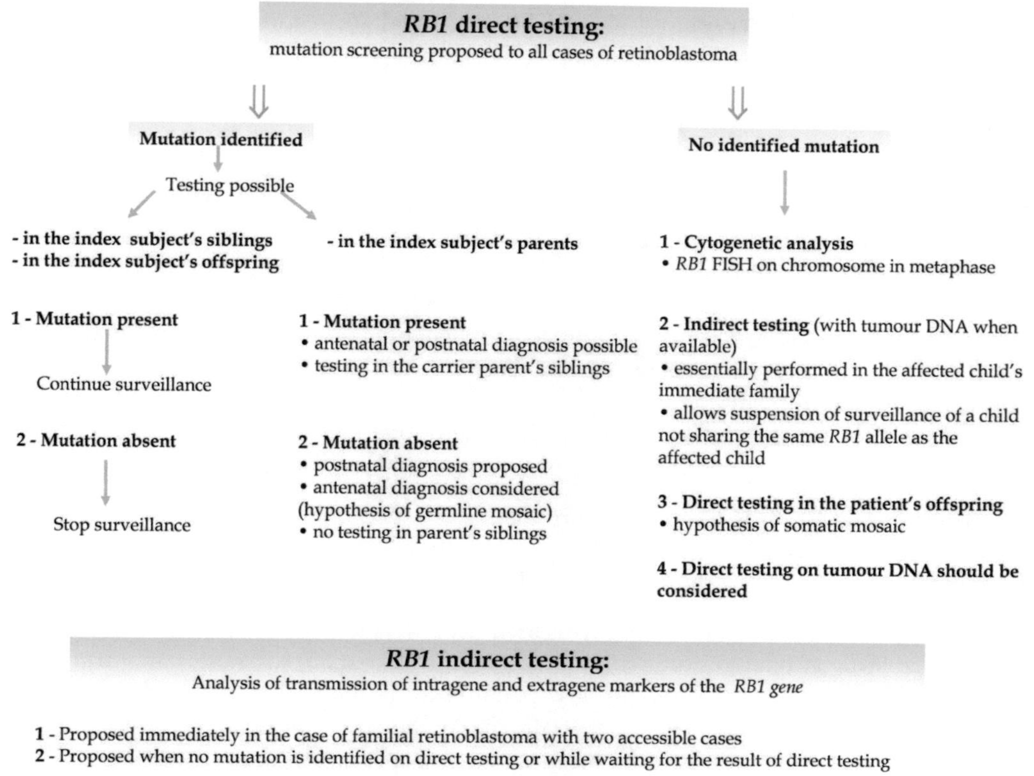

Fig. 2. Clinical management/surveillance

2. In the case of unilateral sporadic retinoblastoma, the genetic counsellor can be more reassuring, as the risk of a genetic predisposition is very low (1% instead of 10%, taking into account a 90% screening sensitivity, see below). However, once again, certain limitations of the techniques used and the risk of somatic mosaic must be kept in mind. It is therefore recommended to continue ophthalmological surveillance in the patient's offspring (Figure 1). However, if the probability of predisposition of a child with unilateral retinoblastoma is only 1%, the risk for his nephews is around 0,00125% or 1/80 000 i.e. lower than in the general population. As a result their ophtalmologic follow-up should be stopped.
3. In familial forms comprising two accessible cases, indirect genetic testing rapidly demonstrates the mutant allele of the *RB1* gene. This method can then be used to detect relatives with the cancer-predisposing allele and allows the possibility of antenatal diagnosis. Indirect molecular genetic testing can also be proposed for families with only one case of retinoblastoma, while waiting for the results of *RB1* screening or when no mutation is detected. The objective in this setting is to suspend surveillance of a child not sharing any *RB1* allele in common with its brother or sister with retinoblastoma, i.e. in one case in four, or even one case in two when loss of heterozygosity is demonstrated in the patient's tumour, designating the remaining allele as the putative predisposing allele. It should be stressed that even when a child shares an allele in common with the patient, the probability that he or she has an *RB1* gene mutation remains very low (Figure 1). However, as a precaution,

ophthalmological surveillance should be continued. Antenatal diagnosis cannot be considered in this particular setting.

2.4 Notes

For a long time, it was considered that all patients with a deleterious *RB1* gene mutation developed retinoblastoma regardless of the type of molecular lesion. However, the risk within a given family has now been clearly established to be heterogeneous, as some members do not develop retinoblastoma, while others develop bilateral retinoblastoma, or even a secondary tumour. The severity of the risk can be evaluated by the disease-eye-ratio (DER), which is a good marker of penetrance and level of expression (Lohmann et al., 1994). The DER is the ratio of the number of eyes affected over the number of carriers within the family. One of the problems of genetic counseling for retinoblastoma is therefore to evaluate the tumour risk for an unborn child with a germline *RB1* gene mutation, hence the importance of developing our knowledge of genotype-phenotype relationships.

In general, subjects with a mutation in the first generation may have an attenuated phenotype due to a possible mosaic. The type of lesion then varies according to the type of mutation (Lohmann&Gallie, 2004, Harbour, 2001, Taylor et al., 2007).

Subjects with a mutation leading to a truncated protein (stop, frameshift) have a high risk, greater than 90%, of bilateral retinoblastoma (mean DER = 1.85). Of note, some truncating mutations in exon 1 may lead to low-penetrance retinoblastoma trough alternative translation initiation (Sanchez-Sanchez et al., 2007). The situation is more complex for the other types of mutations, as discussed below.

Splicing mutations are associated with a lower mean DER (1.5) and, in some cases, with high intrafamily variability with the presence of tumour-free and bilateral cases in the same family. The variability of the DER is mainly due to maintenance of the frame and/or the respect of functional domains. The case of IVS06+1G>T splicing mutation is quite remarkable, as this mutation is supposed to result in a skip of exon 6 out of phase and therefore in the absence of protein, as the truncated messenger is eliminated by Non sense Mediated Decay (NMD) (Holbrook et al., 2004). This mutation is actually associated with an extraordinary variability of intrafamily and interfamily penetrance. The mechanisms proposed to account for this phenomenon are maintenance and therefore translation of the truncated messenger, possibly related to a parental effect (Klutz et al., 2002) or overexpression of the wild-type allele, resulting in a normal level of *RB1* expression (Taylor et al., 2007).

Anomalies of the promoter region are classically associated with variations of the level of expression of the messenger and result in variable but generally low DER.

Missense mutations are very rare. When they do not alter splicing (see above), they can be responsible for a partially functional protein (e.g. R661W), which results in a very low mean DER (0.3), but the possibility of bilateral cases cannot be excluded (Onadim et al., 1992).

Chromosomal rearrangements (deletion or duplication of one or several exons, or even the whole gene) are associated with a variable DER (mean: 1.4), particularly and surprisingly, deletions comprising all of *RB1*, for which the phenotype can vary from no lesion to bilateral retinoblastoma (Albrecht et al., 2005).

The type of mutation therefore affects the type of lesion, but modifying factors influencing splicing, the level of expression and/or cell survival also appear to be involved. As an example, the existence of these genetic modifiers in retinoblastoma have been suspected and searched in the pRB or p53 pathways in which MDM2 is a key regulator of both p53 and pRB catabolism. We have recently demonstrated that the minor allele of *MDM2* that includes a 309T>G transversion (SNP rs2279744) in the *MDM2* promoter is strongly associated under a recessive model with incidence of bilateral or unilateral retinoblastoma among members of retinoblastoma families (Castéra et al., 2010).

In the context of genetic counseling, the possibility of antenatal or even pre-implantation diagnosis can be proposed to couples with a 50% risk of transmitting an *RB1* gene mutation. The situation is obviously more delicate in families presenting an intrafamily heterogeneous risk, which makes genetic counseling more difficult. Although it appears impossible to reassure a parent with no history of retinoblastoma, but carrying an *RB1* mutation about the tumour risk for his/her offspring, it is very difficult to inform this subject about techniques allowing the birth of a mutation-free infant. It is therefore very important to continue the study of these families in order to improve genetic counseling in the context of retinoblastoma.

3. Molecular methods in genetic testing

3.1 Overview

The molecular pathology of *RB1* is very diverse and about 500 distinct germline mutations have been described to date, some of which are listed in two databases managed by Dr Lohmann *(http://RB1-lsdb.d-lohmann.de)* and Dr Pestaña (http://www.es.embnet.org/Services/MolBio/rbgmdb). These mutations occur throughout the coding sequence and in the promoter region with the notable exception of the last 2 exons (figure 3). Most of these

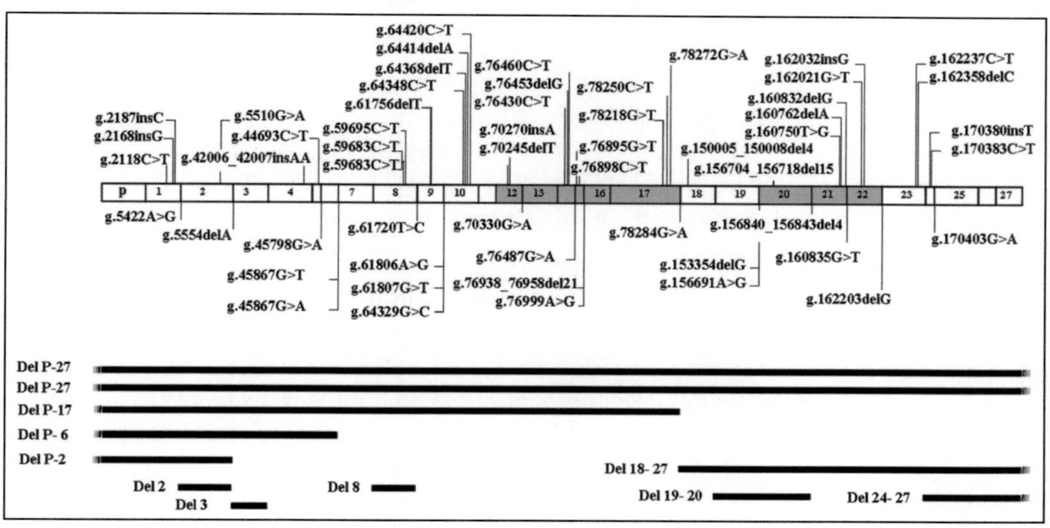

RB1 coding sequence is drawn to scale, and exons shown in grey are part of pocket domains A or B. Large deletions are represented as black lines.

Fig. 3. Pattern of mutations found in a series of 192 retinoblastoma patients (adapted from Houdayer et al., 2004)

mutations are *de novo* mutations. The spectrum of germline mutations mainly comprises nonsense mutations (about 40%), frameshift insertions or deletions of several bases (about 25%), altered splicing (about 20%) and chromosomal rearrangements, i.e. deletions/duplications of one or several exons, or even the entire gene (about 10%). The remaining mutations correspond to rare missense mutations and mutations of the promoter region. Variations of the relative proportions of these mutations have been reported, which can be explained by differences of the population studied, and environmental or stochastic factors, related to the high rate of *de novo* mutations (Dehainault et al., 2004, Alonso et al., 2001). Finally, constitutional inactivation of *RB1* can be due to exceptional cases of chromosomal rearrangements only visible on cytogenetics (e.g. translocations, inversions). These same types of alterations are also found in the tumour, as well as hypermethylation of the promoter region and large chromosomal losses comprising all of *RB1* and flanking regions (Richter et al., 2003).Tumoral events are now systematically searched when the tumor is available.

3.2 Materials

Analysis of the index case, which requires a larger amount of material, must be distinguished from that of relatives, in whom the search for a previously identified mutation requires less material.

3.2.1 Study of the index case

Testing for germline *RB1* gene mutations is classically performed on DNA extracted from whole blood collected on EDTA. Two to 3 µg of genomic DNA are required for screening for point mutations and large mutations on the entire gene. Extraction can be performed with commercial kits or by phenol/chloroform or perchlorate/chloroform or salting out techniques (Johns&Paulus-Thomas, 1989, Miller et al., 1988).

When DNA is used for screening, RNA must also be available due to the frequency of splicing alterations. RNA analysis may be essential to demonstrate the impact of the presumptive mutation identified on genomic DNA. RNA is obtained from a blood sample collected on heparin, Acid Citrate Dextrose (ACD), or EDTA. Lymphoblastoid cell culture is an interesting option, as it provides an infinite source of nucleic acids, but it is expensive and requires cell culture facilities.

Finally, tumour DNA analysis is important for the molecular diagnosis of retinoblastoma. Samples fixed in Bouin's solution cannot be used, as this fixative degrades DNA, and frozen blocks are preferable to paraffin-embedded blocks. When the first-line analysis is performed on the tumour (see below), a sufficient amount of material must be available (2 to 3 µg). A small quantity is sufficient when looking for a known mutation and it is even possible to obtain genetic material by scratching a slide. Tumour DNA can be extracted with commercial kits or phenol/chloroform.

3.2.2 Study of relatives

In this setting, genetic testing is designed to detect a previously identified mutation, and a small quantity of DNA is sufficient (about 50 ng) and can be extracted from buccal cells collected by swabbing, a simple, noninvasive technique. FTA technology (Gaytmenn et al., 2002, Seah et al., 2003) is then the preferred method: swabs are applied onto FTA cards, buccal cells are then lysed and nucleic acids are immobilized and stabilized in the FTA matrix. The paper support is then punched out and the punch is washed and placed in the PCR reaction tube. Alternatively, buccal cells can be extracted from the swab by using standard commercial kits.

3.3 Methods

There are two types of diagnostic genetic molecular testing: direct testing and indirect testing.

3.3.1 Direct testing

Direct testing consists of looking for a germline alteration of the *RB1* gene indicative of a predisposition to retinoblastoma. The first study performed in a family is time-consuming and generally takes several months. In contrast, when testing is performed to detect a mutation already identified in the family, targeted screening of the previously identified mutation takes only a few days. Direct testing is essentially performed on blood samples. It is good practice to verify the presence of a mutation on two DNA samples obtained independently: two blood samples taken at two different times, or a blood test and a buccal swab.

Direct testing can also be performed on the tumour. This screening can be very useful in bilateral cases in which no mutation is detected on leukocytes, but also for unilateral forms, as identification of a mutation only in the tumour would be very useful for genetic counselling, eliminating the risk of recurrence in siblings and cousins (but not in the offspring). Testing of tumour DNA is obviously subject to availability of material, i.e. enucleation.

The complexity of the mutational spectrum of the *RB1* gene requires analysis of the entire coding sequence and promoter region by several complementary techniques (see DNA methylation analysis).

3.3.1.1 Detection of point mutations

Point mutations are usually investigated by Denaturing High Performance Liquid Chromatography (Xiao&Oefner, 2001, Dehainault et al., 2004) and/or direct DNA sequencing (Richter et al., 2003), or even Denaturing Gradient Gel Electrophoresis (which is more complicated to perform) (Fodde&Losekoot, 1994) or Single Strand Conformational Polymorphism (low sensitivity) (Orita et al., 1989). Recently, we have adapted a novel HDA method (Houdayer et al., 2010) called Enhanced Mismatch Mutation Analysis (EMMA).

Regardless of the technique used, the gene is cut into amplicons corresponding to the exon sequence and intron/exon junctions in order to detect any abnormalities of splicing consensus sequences which can have major functional consequences.

DHPLC is an adaptation of high performance liquid chromatography for DNA applications, used for the detection of point mutations. It is based on the principle of physical separation, under denaturing conditions, of various DNA fragments in a mobile phase by differential retention on a solid phase composed of a DNA column. DHPLC has a high sensitivity, making it a very useful tool in retinoblastoma for the study of tumours or mosaics, which are not uncommon. DHPLC is able to detect less than 20% of the minority allelic species, which corresponds to the accepted limit for sequencing. The limitations of DHPLC depend on the base composition of the DNA fragment studied (see "Notes" section).

EMMA is based on the use of innovative matrices increasing the electrophoretic mobility differences between homoduplex and heteroduplex. DNA Sensitivity is further improved by using nucleosides as additives to enhance single-base substitution detection. Nucleosides are expected to interact with mismatched bases of heteroduplexes, thereby increasing mobility differences with homoduplexes. Moreover, this method, in combination with adapted semiquantitative PCR conditions, can be used to simultaneously detect point mutations and large-scale rearrangement in a single run (Weber et al., 2006, Weber et al., 2007). This feature, combined with the use of a single set of separation conditions for all fragments and with the multiplexing capability of the method, leads to a considerable simplification and cost reduction compared to previous methods (Caux-Moncoutier et al., 2010).

Direct sequencing is the second option and is considered to be the reference technique. However, its performances are highly dependent on the apparatus, chemistry, polymers and software used. A study comparing DHPLC and direct sequencing for BRCA1 analysis concluded on a similar detection rate for the two techniques (Alonso et al., 2001).

Direct testing is also performed on RNA to characterize any abnormal splicing. Classically, after extraction of RNA and RT PCR, the cDNA region surrounding the putative anomaly is amplified to demonstrate abnormal transcripts. The instability of messenger RNA carrying a premature stop codon, or NMD (Holbrook et al., 2004), constitutes a real problem in diagnostic molecular genetics and is discussed in the "Notes" section.

3.3.1.2 Detection of chromosomal rearrangements

Chromosomal rearrangements, i.e. deletion/duplication of one or several exons, cannot be detected by the techniques used to detect point mutations because the mutant allele is masked by the wild-type allele, as the retinoblastoma susceptibility gene segregates according to an autosomal dominant mode.

Specific gene assay techniques must be used in order to distinguish 2 copies of the target (wild-type status), one copy (deletion) or 3 copies (duplication). Semiquantitative techniques, such as Quantitative Multiplex PCR of Short fluorescent Fragments (QMPSF), Multiplex PCR/liquid chromatography assay (MP/LC) (Duponchel et al., 2001, Dehainault et al., 2004), and Multiplex Ligation Probe Amplification (MLPA) (Schouten et al., 2002) or quantitative techniques, i.e. real-time PCR, are used. QMPSF is a technique allowing simultaneous, semiquantitative amplification of several exons; the intensity of the signal obtained therefore depends on the number of copies of the gene of interest in the matrix DNA. After amplification of the exons followed by separation of the PCR products obtained by electrophoresis, the patient electrophoretograms are compared to those of normal and mutant controls. The signal intensity in the various samples is then evaluated and deletions of one or several amplicons are revealed by a 50% reduction of the corresponding peak(s). Data can be exported to an Excel spreadsheet and analysed by a macro. The advantage of

QMPSF and other semiquantitative multiplex PCR approaches is their high throughput and the small number of analytical steps, which is always appreciated in the diagnostic setting.

Another widely used semiquantitative technique, MLPA, is based on a step of hybridization of specific probes, fitted with a universal tail, and corresponding to the exons to be examined. The quantity of probe hybridized is therefore proportional to the quantity of target. After hybridization and ligation, probes are then amplified by PCR with a set of universal primers and PCR products are separated be capillary electrophoresis. Once again, the signal intensity, compared to that of normal and mutant controls, is used to detect chromosomal rearrangements. Despite a much higher multiplexing capacity, the throughput of MLPA is lower than that of semiquantitative multiplex PCR approaches due to an additional analytical step (ligation), but the advantage of this technique is that it is available in the form of ready-for-use kits for many genes including *RB1*.

These two approaches have similar performances and the choice between the two therefore depends on the user's priorities.

Real-time PCR techniques are particularly suitable for gene assays. They are based on either i) incorporation of a free fluorophore (typically SYBR Green) into the forming strands, which generates an increase in the intensity of fluorescence with the number of copies produced. The sensitivity of these techniques is enhanced by the use of fluorophore-labelled specific probes. Unfortunately, they have a low throughput, limited by the number of fluorophores available and are therefore not widely used for screening, especially as this low throughput is not justified by the gain in sensitivity.

An approach combining the search for point mutations and chromosomal rearrangements achieves a germline *RB1* gene mutation detection rate of about 90% among patients with bilateral retinoblastoma (Richter et al., 2003). The mutations that are not detected are probably deep intronic anomalies, responsible for alternative splicing defects that are not detected because they are situated outside of the zones usually studied (Dehainault et al., 2007). They can also correspond to mosaics, which cannot be detected on circulating leukocytes (see "Notes" section).

3.3.1.3 DNA methylation analysis

Hypermethylation of the promoter region is a common mutational event found in tumor (Richter et al., 2003). Hypermethylation of the promoter are investigated by bisulfite analysis followed either by sequencing, by methylation-specific PCR or by a quantitative analysis of methylated allele using specific Taqman® probes (De La Rosa-Velazquez et al., 2007, Richter et al., 2003, Zeschnigk et al., 2004). Alternatively, tumor DNA can be digested using methylation sensitive enzyme (CfoI as an example), followed by PCR amplification of the promoter and agarose gel electrophoresis or followed by a semiquantitative technique such as QMPSF (Taylor et al., 2007).

3.3.2 Indirect testing

Indirect testing is based on amplification of polymorphic markers of the *RB1* locus. Analysis of polymorphic genetic markers localized in and around the *RB1* gene in an affected child and his parents is designed to identify the *RB1* allele carrying or putatively carrying a predisposition to retinoblastoma. Indirect tests are very useful in familial cases, when samples are available for at least two cases of retinoblastoma, to identify the allele of the *RB1* gene common to affected cases, i.e. to determine the allele that carries the mutation, even when the mutation has not been demonstrated directly. In non-familial forms, reconstitution of the affected child's alleles reveals the two alleles putatively associated with an alteration of the *RB1* gene. Tumour DNA studies (when available) reveal loss of an allele in 65% of cases and consequently allow identification of the remaining allele, i.e. potentially carrying a germline mutation. The indirect approach is technically simple and rapid, but nevertheless requires testing of the affected child, the parents, and possibly other relatives.

3.3.3 Cytogenetic analysis

Cytogenetic analysis comprises a standard karyotype and analysis of the *RB1* gene by FISH or CGH-array. The development of molecular genetic studies has considerably limited the applications of cytogenetics and its only first-line indication is for karyotyping in a child with mental retardation or a malformative syndrome associated with retinoblastoma. However, it remains useful for the detection of translocations and mosaic deletions and can help to estimate the size of very large deletions. It therefore reveals certain rare situations.

High density CGH array may be useful for fine mapping of deletion breakpoints in a context of a contiguous gene syndrome (Mitter et al., 2011)

3.4 Notes

3.4.1 General problems

3.4.1.1 GC-rich regions

The 5′ part of the *RB1* gene (promoter and exon 1) is particularly rich in GC, which can make it difficult to analyse, for the detection of both point mutations and rearrangements. Due to the high degree of similarity of the amplified region, nonspecific intrastrand base pairing tends to occur during PCR, resulting in nonspecific PCR. Consequently, some teams do not analyse this region, which makes the analysis incomplete, as mutations of the promoter region and exon 1 have been well documented. We have resolved these problems by the addition of dimethylsulfoxyde (DMSO) to the reaction medium.

3.4.1.2 Mosaics

The existence of somatic mosaics in retinoblastoma raises a major problem for molecular diagnosis, as the mutant clone may be below the limit of detection of the technique used, or may even be absent from the cells studied. We have identified a deleterious *RB1* mutation from a blood sample of an affected child in whom tumour material was not available. Surprisingly, this mutation was detected in a very small percentage (estimated at 10%) of buccal cells. DHPLC is particularly useful in this context because of its high sensitivity, but characterization of the anomaly by sequencing remains problematical and requires specific techniques (fraction collector, specific primers, cloning, etc.).

3.4.1.3 Abnormalities of splicing

Splicing abnormalities represent 20% of the mutational spectrum of *RB1* and are therefore important to characterize. Unfortunately, the instability of messenger RNA carrying a premature stop codon means that the truncated messenger RNA is below the limit of detection and only the wild-type transcript will be visible, wrongly suggesting the absence of an anomaly. This problem can sometimes be resolved by using translation inhibitors, such as puromycin, which eliminate NMD and therefore improve detection of the truncated messenger RNA (Andreutti-Zaugg et al., 1997).

Some deep intronic anomalies, responsible for alternative splicing, are probably not detected because they are situated outside the zones routinely studied. Systematic RNA analysis would be required to demonstrate these anomalies. This approach, unsuitable for routine testing, is nevertheless used in the case of failure of other techniques in situations of highly probable predisposition, such as cases of bilateral and/or familial retinoblastoma with no identified mutation (Dehainault et al., 2007).

3.4.2 Detection of point mutations by DHPLC

DHPLC is a sensitive and reliable technique for the detection of point mutations. However, its efficacy is subject to the availability of specific, high-yield PCR and rigorous system quality control, as the gradient drift can impair the quality of testing by modifying retention times and, much more insidiously, loss of calibration, even minimal, of the oven can be responsible for a drastic reduction of resolution for certain amplicons, generating false-negative results. It is therefore essential to ensure the integrity of the system each day by using control samples. Control samples should generate slight modifications of the profile, which can therefore only be detected with an optimally functioning system. The limitations of this method, which depend on the base composition of the DNA fragment studied, must be kept in mind. For example, despite all of our efforts, we have not been able to obtain reliable results for exon 8 of *RB1*, which must be sequenced as first-line procedure (Dehainault et al., 2004). This point has also been emphasized by P. Oefner, the inventor of DHPLC (Sivakumaran et al., 2005).

3.4.3 Detection of chromosomal rearrangements by semiquantitative techniques

MLPA or semiquantitative multiplex PCR techniques (such as QMPSF) are robust techniques, but highly dependent on the quality of the DNA studied. Degraded DNA will be responsible for loss of proportionality between signal intensity and copy number, particularly for large fragments, making the analysis uninterpretable. Contamination of DNA by phenol will have an even greater effect, because it generates a random fluctuation of signal intensity. Phenol-free extraction techniques should therefore be preferred (perchlorate/chloroform or column-based commercial kits) or a system ensuring the absence of contamination by phenol such as the gel lock extraction system, which uses a gel-barrier system (Eppendorf®).

It is also essential to adjust all DNA samples studied to a suitable working concentration, classically 50 ng/µl. If the DNA concentration is too high, for example, the proportionality between signal intensity and copy number will be lost, particularly for small fragments. DNA calibration can be performed with: i) a tube spectrophotometer (unsuitable for large series); ii) the NanoDrop from NanoDrop technologies (which has the advantage of tracing the spectrum of the sample); or iii) a plate reader (rapid, but reading at only one wavelength at a time). In our experience, the use of fluorescent dyes for the assay, such as PicoGreen (Molecular Probes), is unnecessary for these applications.

Finally, buccal swabs are poorly adapted to these analyses, including for the search of a mutation already identified in a relative, as DNA is often present in a low concentration and difficult to calibrate for FTA samples.

Due to the importance of quality/quantity/calibration of DNA solutions, laboratories often prefer to extract DNA locally and therefore ask to receive whole blood.

A classical trap in the interpretation of these techniques concerns the false-positive results generated by a PCR primer mismatch. Each deletion of a single exon must therefore be systematically checked by another technique and/or by shifting the primers (long range PCR, RNA studies, real-time PCR, for example). Finally, duplication of an isolated exon is the most difficult case to characterize. The ideal situation is therefore to have a duplicated control of the entire *RB1*, for example DNA from a case of trisomy 13.

4. Conclusion

Finally, we recommend a systematic *RB1* molecular screening to all retinoblastoma patients as part of routine clinical care. Emphasis is placed on close collaboration between laboratory staff and clinicians to ensure effective communication and therefore adequate genetic counseling.

5. Acknowledgments

We thank Christine Levy, Livia Lumbroso, Jean Michon, Isabelle Aerts, Gudrun Schleiermacher, Daniel Orbach, Hélène Pacquement, Jérôme Couturier, Catherine Dehainault, Dorothée Michaux for participating in Institut Curie Retinoblastoma pluridisciplinary group. This work was supported by grants from the Programme Incitatif et Coopératif sur le Rétinoblastome (Institut Curie) and RETINOSTOP.

6. References

Abramson DH, Mendelsohn ME, Servodidio CA, et al. (1998). Familial retinoblastoma: where and when? *Acta Ophthalmol Scand* 76, pp 334-8

Albrecht P, Ansperger-Rescher B, Schuler A, et al. (2005). Spectrum of gross deletions and insertions in the RB1 gene in patients with retinoblastoma and association with phenotypic expression. *Hum Mutat* 26, pp 437-45

Alonso J, Garcia-Miguel P, Abelairas J, et al. (2001). Spectrum of germline RB1 gene mutations in Spanish retinoblastoma patients: Phenotypic and molecular epidemiological implications. *Hum Mutat* 17, pp 412-22

Andreutti-Zaugg C, Scott RJIggo R. (1997). Inhibition of nonsense-mediated messenger RNA decay in clinical samples facilitates detection of human MSH2 mutations with an in vivo fusion protein assay and conventional techniques. *Cancer Res* 57, pp 3288-93

Baud O, Cormier-Daire V, Lyonnet S, et al. (1999). Dysmorphic phenotype and neurological impairment in 22 retinoblastoma patients with constitutional cytogenetic 13q deletion. *Clin Genet* 55, pp 478-82

Bremner R, Chen D, Pacal M, et al. (2004). The RB protein family in retinal development and retinoblastoma: new insights from new mouse models. *Dev Neurosci* 26, pp 417-34,

Castera L, Sabbagh A, Dehainault C, et al. (2010). MDM2 as a modifier gene in retinoblastoma. *J Natl Cancer Inst* 102, pp 1805-8

Caux-Moncoutier V, Castera L, Tirapo C, et al. (2010). EMMA, a cost- and time-effective diagnostic method for simultaneous detection of point mutations and large-scale genomic rearrangements: application to BRCA1 and BRCA2 in 1,525 patients. *Hum Mutat*,

Chau BNWang JY. (2003). Coordinated regulation of life and death by RB. *Nat Rev Cancer* 3, pp 130-8,

Classon MHarlow E. (2002). The retinoblastoma tumour suppressor in development and cancer. *Nat Rev Cancer* 2, pp 910-7

Comings DE. (1973). A general theory of carcinogenesis. *Proc Natl Acad Sci U S A* 70, pp 3324-8

De La Rosa-Velazquez IA, Rincon-Arano H, Benitez-Bribiesca L, et al. (2007). Epigenetic regulation of the human retinoblastoma tumor suppressor gene promoter by CTCF. *Cancer Res* 67, pp 2577-85

Dehainault C, Lauge A, Caux-Moncoutier V, et al. (2004). Multiplex PCR/liquid chromatography assay for detection of gene rearrangements: application to RB1 gene. *Nucleic Acids Res* 32, pp e139

Dehainault C, Michaux D, Pages-Berhouet S, et al. (2007). A deep intronic mutation in the RB1 gene leads to intronic sequence exonisation. *Eur J Hum Genet* 15, pp 473-7,

Draper GJ, Sanders BMKingston JE. (1986). Second primary neoplasms in patients with retinoblastoma. *Br J Cancer* 53, pp 661-71

Duponchel C, Di Rocco C, Cicardi M, et al. (2001). Rapid detection by fluorescent multiplex PCR of exon deletions and duplications in the C1 inhibitor gene of hereditary angioedema patients. *Hum Mutat* 17, pp 61-70

Fletcher O, Easton D, Anderson K, et al. (2004). Lifetime risks of common cancers among retinoblastoma survivors. *J Natl Cancer Inst* 96, pp 357-63,

Fodde RLosekoot M. (1994). Mutation detection by denaturing gradient gel electrophoresis (DGGE). *Hum Mutat* 3, pp 83-94

Friend SH, Bernards R, Rogelj S, et al. (1986). A human DNA segment with properties of the gene that predisposes to retinoblastoma and osteosarcoma. *Nature* 323, pp 643-6

Gaytmenn R, Hildebrand DP, Sweet D, et al. (2002). Determination of the sensitivity and specificity of sibship calculations using AmpF lSTR Profiler Plus. *Int J Legal Med* 116, pp 161-4

Harbour JW. (2001). Molecular basis of low-penetrance retinoblastoma. *Arch Ophthalmol* 119, pp 1699-704

Holbrook JA, Neu-Yilik G, Hentze MW, et al. (2004). Nonsense-mediated decay approaches the clinic. *Nat Genet* 36, pp 801-8

Houdayer C, Gauthier-Villars M, Lauge A, et al. (2004). Comprehensive screening for constitutional RB1 mutations by DHPLC and QMPSF. *Hum Mutat* 23, pp 193-202

Houdayer C, Moncoutier V, Champ J, et al. (2010). Enhanced mismatch mutation analysis: simultaneous detection of point mutations and large scale rearrangements by capillary electrophoresis, application to BRCA1 and BRCA2. *Methods Mol Biol* 653, pp 147-80

Johns MB, Jr.Paulus-Thomas JE. (1989). Purification of human genomic DNA from whole blood using sodium perchlorate in place of phenol. *Anal Biochem* 180, pp 276-8

Klutz M, Brockmann DLohmann DR. (2002). A parent-of-origin effect in two families with retinoblastoma is associated with a distinct splice mutation in the RB1 gene. *Am J Hum Genet* 71, pp 174-9

Knudson AG, Jr. (1971). Mutation and cancer: statistical study of retinoblastoma. *Proc Natl Acad Sci U S A* 68, pp 820-3

Lele KP, Penrose LSStallard HB. (1963). Chromosome Deletion in a Case of Retinoblastoma. *Ann Hum Genet* 27, pp 171-4

Lohmann DR, Brandt B, Hopping W, et al. (1994). Distinct RB1 gene mutations with low penetrance in hereditary retinoblastoma. *Hum Genet* 94, pp 349-54

Lohmann DRGallie BL. (2004). Retinoblastoma: revisiting the model prototype of inherited cancer. *Am J Med Genet C Semin Med Genet* 129, pp 23-8

Miller SA, Dykes DDPolesky HF. (1988). A simple salting out procedure for extracting DNA from human nucleated cells. *Nucleic Acids Res* 16, pp 1215

Mitter D, Ullmann R, Muradyan A, et al. (2011). Genotype-phenotype correlations in patients with retinoblastoma and interstitial 13q deletions. *Eur J Hum Genet* 19, pp 947-958, 1476-5438 (Electronic) 1018-4813 (Linking).

Moll AC, Imhof SM, Bouter LM, et al. (1996). Second primary tumors in patients with hereditary retinoblastoma: a register-based follow-up study, 1945-1994. *Int J Cancer* 67, pp 515-9

Moll AC, Imhof SM, Meeteren AY, et al. (2000). At what age could screening for familial retinoblastoma be stopped? A register based study 1945-98. *Br J Ophthalmol* 84, pp 1170-2

Musarella MAGallie BL. (1987). A simplified scheme for genetic counseling in retinoblastoma. *J Pediatr Ophthalmol Strabismus* 24, pp 124-5

Onadim Z, Hogg A, Baird PN, et al. (1992). Oncogenic point mutations in exon 20 of the RB1 gene in families showing incomplete penetrance and mild expression of the retinoblastoma phenotype. *Proc Natl Acad Sci U S A* 89, pp 6177-81

Orita M, Suzuki Y, Sekiya T, et al. (1989). Rapid and sensitive detection of point mutations and DNA polymorphisms using the polymerase chain reaction. *Genomics* 5, pp 874-9

Richter S, Vandezande K, Chen N, et al. (2003). Sensitive and efficient detection of RB1 gene mutations enhances care for families with retinoblastoma. *Am J Hum Genet* 72, pp 253-69,

Sanchez-Sanchez F, Ramirez-Castillejo C, Weekes DB, et al. (2007). Attenuation of disease phenotype through alternative translation initiation in low-penetrance retinoblastoma. *Hum Mutat* 28, pp 159-67,

Schouten JP, McElgunn CJ, Waaijer R, et al. (2002). Relative quantification of 40 nucleic acid sequences by multiplex ligation-dependent probe amplification. *Nucleic Acids Res* 30, pp e57,

Seah LH, Jeevan NH, Othman MI, et al. (2003). STR Data for the AmpFlSTR Identifiler loci in three ethnic groups (Malay, Chinese, Indian) of the Malaysian population. *Forensic Sci Int* 138, pp 134-7,

Sivakumaran TA, Shen P, Wall DP, et al. (2005). Conservation of the RB1 gene in human and primates. *Hum Mutat* 25, pp 396-409,

Taylor M, Dehainault C, Desjardins L, et al. (2007). Genotype-phenotype correlations in hereditary familial retinoblastoma. *Hum Mutat* 28, pp 284-93,

Weber J, Looten R, Houdayer C, et al. (2006). Improving sensitivity of electrophoretic heteroduplex analysis using nucleosides as additives: Application to the breast cancer predisposition gene BRCA2. *Electrophoresis* 27, pp 1444-52,

Weber J, Miserere S, Champ J, et al. (2007). High-throughput simultaneous detection of point mutations and large-scale rearrangements by CE. *Electrophoresis* 28, pp 4282-8,

Xiao WOefner PJ. (2001). Denaturing high-performance liquid chromatography: A review. *Hum Mutat* 17, pp 439-74,

Zeschnigk M, Bohringer S, Price EA, et al. (2004). A novel real-time PCR assay for quantitative analysis of methylated alleles (QAMA): analysis of the retinoblastoma locus. *Nucleic Acids Res* 32, pp e125,

Zhu L. (2005). Tumour suppressor retinoblastoma protein Rb: a transcriptional regulator. *Eur J Cancer* 41, pp 2415-27,

Part 2

Epidemiology

5

Epidemiology of Retinoblastoma

Wilson O. Akhiwu[1] and Alex P. Igbe[2]
[1]*Histopathology Department, University of Benin Teaching Hospital, Benin City, Edo State*
[2]*Histopathology Department, Ambrose Alli University Ekpoma, Edo State*
Nigeria

1. Introduction

It is widely acknowledged that cancers are disorders of cell growth and behavior and that its cause has to be defined at cellular levels. However, studies have shown that the cause of cancer can be deduced from a study of its epidemiology. Sir Percival Pott is credited with linking chemicals to causing cancer when he observed astutely that Chimney sweeps, because of their chronic exposure to sooth, were prone to scrotal cancers. Subsequently, the Danish Chimney sweeps guild ruled that its members must have their bath daily and this prevented the problem.[1] Prior to this, John Hill had linked nasal polyps to "immoderate use of snuff". Epidemiology has also contributed in linking cervical cancer to human papilloma viruses and radiation to different cancers[1]. It is also important for the purposes of health planning and allocation of resources to know the distribution of any particular disease.

Retinoblastoma, an embryonal tumour originating from retinal cells, is reputed to be the commonest intraocular malignancy in children. Currently, retinoblastoma is the most common solid tumour in children after brain/nervous system tumours and lymphomas in the United Kingdom.[2] Kramarova and Stiller also reported a similar pattern among American children.[3] In Nigeria, retinoblastoma is second only to lymphoma in most studies[4,5,6] and third in some series.[7] Report from other African countries shows that this tumour is the second most common childhood solid tumour.[8]

2. Age distribution

Age has an important influence on the likelihood of beings afflicted with cancer. The incidence of cancer rises with advancing age and most cases occur in people aged 55years and above. The age related rising incidence may be explained by the accumulation of mutations associated with the emergence of cancers. Most cases of retinoblastoma, however, occur in childhood with over 90% being diagnosed before five years of age; only 24 cases have been reported in adults aged between 20years and 74 years.[9] The worldwide incidence rate of retinoblastoma for children aged 0-4years varies from 3.4% per million in Bulgaria[10] to a very high 42.5 per million in Mali.[11] Incidence rates vary greatly in some regions while it varies only slightly in some other regions (table 1).

Region	Incidence
Australia	1.4
Belgium	1
Canada	2
Croatia	0.7
Czech Republic	0.7
Denmark	1.3
Estonia	1.5
Finland	1.1
France	1.6
Germany	2.3
1celand	1.1
Ireland	1.0
Italy	1.4
Latvia	0.2
Lithuania	1.4
Malta	1.9
New Zealand	2.2
Norway	0.7
Poland	0.6
Portugal	3.6
Russia	1.3
Slovakia	1.5
Slovenia	1.0
Sweden	3.5
Switzerland	1.7
The Netherlands	1.2
United Kingdom	1.3
United States White	1.4
United States Hispanic	1.4
Yugoslavia	o.2

Table 1. Average incidence for whites in the United States and Nations with greater than 85% White population *(adapted from J Pediatr Ophthalmol Strabismus 2009 ;46: 288-293)*

A large study in the USA[12] covering a 30year period from1975 - 2004 using the Surveillance Epidemiology and End Results (SEER) programme database of the National Cancer Institute found 658 of retinoblastoma cases over the period. The overall mean adjusted incidence was 11.3 for males and 12.4 for females. Seventy two per cent (72%) were unilateral while 27% were bilateral. In 1% of cases the laterality was unknown. With increasing age at diagnosis, the bilateral tumours decreased significantly. However, the percentage of unilateral tumours increased with increasing age at diagnosis. The overall incidence of retinoblastoma also reduced with increasing age (Figure 1). Bilateral new cases are not seen after the age of 3years. The peak age of presentation for both bilateral and unilateral retinoblastoma in the USA is before one year of age. Thereafter, the incidence reduced steeply with age. Only 4.3% of new cases of retinoblastoma were seen between the ages of 5-9years in this study.

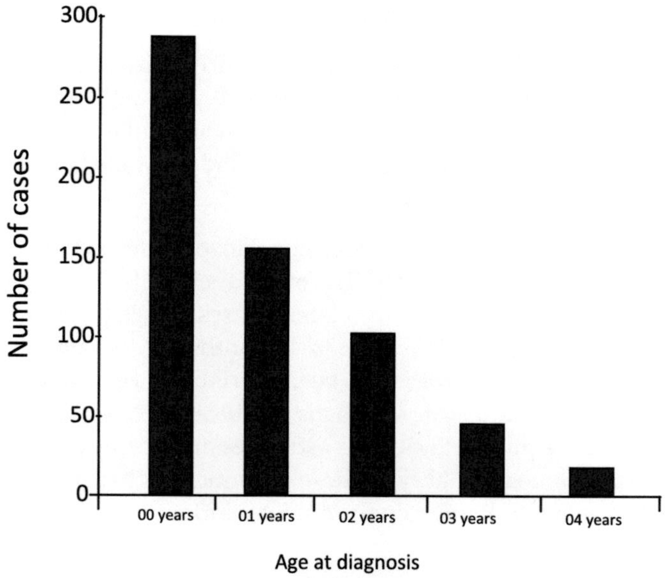

Fig. 1. Distribution of retinoblastoma by age at diagnosis (*Adapted from Br J Ophthalmol 2009; 93: 21-23*)

Another work in the USA[13] from 1993 to 1997 using data from the international agency for cancer found a rate incidence of 4.4 per million for white children with most of the other findings similar to the findings by Broaddus et al.[12]

In Great Britain,[14] retinoblastoma affects approximately 1 in 20000 children. The bilateral cases make up 36% of the total cases. In this study in the UK, using the National Registry for Childhood Tumours (NRCT), the peak incidence was in children below one year, similar to findings in USA studies. After the age of one year, the incidence reduced steadily. Children older than four years made up less than 5% of new cases. The peak age for unilateral cases is in the two year age group while that of bilateral cases is before the first birthday. British studies have shown that unilaterality does not rule out heredity. In this series reported by MacCarthy et al, almost 11% of the unilateral retinoblastoma was heritable cases. All the bilateral cases are usually heritable.

A Swedish and Finish[15] study covering 1958 to 1998 using data from cancer registries and corresponding national referral centers for retinoblastoma found 0-13 and 0-10 new cases per year in Sweden and Finland respectively. The incidence rates per million children under

5years in Sweden and Finland was 11.8 and 11.2 respectively. In this study 90-96% of all retinoblastomas were diagnosed in children less than 5 years.

In Pakistani studies,[16] between 1999 and 2002 found 70 retinoblastoma cases, with 93% of them in children below 5years; 67% of the cases were bilateral. Bilateral cases became less prevalent with increasing age while the unilateral cases peaked in the 2-3year age group with a gradual decline thereafter. The mean at presentation is 28.17 months, unilateral cases having a mean age of 31.81 months. In China,[17] a study covering 1957 to 2006 found that 1234 eyes were enucleated due to retinoblastoma in a specialist eye hospital. The mean age was 2.8years with a range of 1 month to 14years. Bilateral tumours accounted 2.4% of cases, an interesting finding. This was attributed to the nature of their study.

In South Africa,[18] a study by Freedman and Goldberg in 1976 covering a 20-year period in a specialist eye Hospital found 71 cases out of which 82% were unilateral and the other 18% bilateral. The average of the unilateral cases was 3½ years while while for the bilateral, it was 3years, much higher than the findings in western industrialized countries; 80% of cases were diagnosed before the age of 4years.

In a Congolese[19] study carried out in a teaching Hospital on Congolese blacks over a 58month period found 21% bilateral cases. The mean age for all cases was 2.94years with a 4months to 6years. The mean age for the bilateral cases was 1.12years. The mean age in other African studies ranged from 24months to 44months.[20,21,22,23] The relatively advanced age of presentation in African series has been attributed very late presentation. The African patients may seek alternative means of healing before coming to hospital. Incidence studies in Africa put the incidence estimates at 20 cases per million in Malawi[24] and 9.3 per million in Guinea Conakry.[25] These are much higher than rates in USA. This has been attributed to some unknown environmental influences and the higher birth rates in Africa.

In Nigeria, retinoblastoma is the commonest childhood intraocular malignancy with a mean age at presentation of 29 months. For bilateral retinoblastoma which accounted for 13% of cases, the mean age at presentation was younger at 15 months.[26]

3. Sex distribution

Most studies from different parts of the world suggest no sex discrepancy in the incidence of retinoblastoma. In the USA, studies by different workers[12,13] have found an age adjusted incidence of 11.3 for males and 12.4 for females suggesting a mild female predominance. This difference however was not significant.

In Mexico,[27] a study carried out in sixteen centers over a 5-year period showed a non significant mild male predominance of 1.1: 1.0 for all the cases seen. These studies do not show any breakdown of the sex distribution between the age groups and between the unilateral, bilateral and other types of retinoblastoma.

In Great Britain, the study by MacCarthy et al[14] showed that overall, males and females had no difference in the distribution of retinoblastoma for all ages. However, for the 0-1year age group in bilateral retinoblastoma category, there is a 1.1: 1.0 male predominance. For the 1-2 year age group, the male: female predominance for the bilateral tumours is 1.3: 1.0 while for the 2-3year age group, it is 2.2: 1.0. All other age groups showed no significant M:F difference in the incidence of bilateral retinoblastoma. For bilateral tumours for all ages, the M:F ratio 1.3: 1.0.

In Pakistan, Arif Mohamed et al[16] found an equal sex distribution for retinoblastomas in childhood. There was also no gender difference between the unilateral and the bilateral cases.

In China,[17] between the years 1977 to 1996, there was a marked male predominance of 3: 2 and an insignificant overall male predominance of 2.6: 2.0. As in many other studies, the sex distribution between the unilateral and bilateral tumours is not stated.

In Southern Africa studies,[18] there is a marked male predominance over females (3:1) in the bilateral cases. However, for the unilateral cases, the ratio of males to females is 1.2: 1.0. For the1-2year age group, the M: F ratio is about 2: 1. Overall however the M: F ratio is 4:3.

Studies from Congo[19] show a M: F predominance for all cases of retinoblastoma seen over a 6year period to be 2:1. Some other African studies show a male: female ratio of 1.1[20,21]

In Ilorin, Nigeria,[26] there was a mild female predominance of 1.2: 1 overall. The mean age for females and males was also not significant at 31 months and 27 months respectively. However, Akang et al[20] from Ibadan, Nigeria reported a female predominance of 3:2.

4. Geographical/racial distribution

Retinoblastoma has a worldwide distribution. It has been reported from different parts of the world. Because the pathogenesis of retinoblastoma is linked with genetic alterations in the tumour suppressor Rb gene on chromosome 13q14, one would expect a racial variation.

A study by Krishna et al[28] covering a 7year period between 1993 and 1997 and using data from International agency for Research on Cancer, a comparison of the racial and geographic incidence patterns of retinoblastoma in North America, South America, Oceania and Eroupe was carried out. This, to our knowledge, is the most comprehensive that attempts to find a racial and geographic pattern in the incidence of retinoblastomas. This work found a higher incidence of retinoblastoma in Hispanics in the USA than in white children in 3 areas- Los Angeles, San Francisco and New Mexico. However, when adjustments were made and comparison with White population was made, there was no significant difference. This was interpreted to mean that retinoblastoma was similar in White and Hispanic populations in the United States. However, Pendergrass and Davis[12] and Howe et al[29] had found higher rates in Hispanic population over the White population. The consensus, however, is that the perceived difference can be attributed to confounding factors such as cancer registration practices or number of cases. In this study, the rate of retinoblastoma in whites in Europe was found to be the same as in Whites in USA. There was also no significant difference in the incidence in White populations in Oceania and USA. It was only the rates in Portugal and Sweden that were significantly higher than rates in the US Whites. This was attributed to cancer reporting practices[30]. The rates in Canada were similar to that in USA. The Broaddus et al study[12] in USA also showed no significant difference between Whites and Blacks in the USA.

Comparing the incidence of retinoblastoma in Africans with that of other advanced countries is difficult because calculating rates in Africans countries is fraught with problems. However, rates of up to 20 per million children under five[24] 9.3 per million age standardized in Guinea Conakry[25] have been noted. These would suggest that the rates are much higher in Africa than the rest of the world. This has been attributed to ignorance, poor health facilities and high birth rates. What, however, is certain is that African retinoblastomas are diagnosed at a significantly later age than in the advanced world.

5. Summary

Retinoblastoma is a childhood cancer with 90% diagnosed before the age five years. Only 24 cases have been reported in adults between 20-74 years worldwide. Unilateral cases are commoner than bilateral cases in a ratio of 2.7: 1. With increasing age at diagnosis, unilateral cases increased significantly while the bilateral cases decreased significantly. However, the overall incidence of retinoblastoma decreases with advancing age. The peak age of presentation is before the age of one year in advanced countries but between the ages of two and three years in Africa due to late presentation. Although many studies show a mild female predominance, this is not significant. However, some European studies note a significant male predominance for bilateral tumours and retinoblastoma diagnosed in the two to three year age group.

The incidence rate varies worldwide with higher levels in Africa and much lower levels in Europe. However, in multiracial countries like the USA, no significant difference between races was found

6. References

[1] Cotran R S, Kumar V, Collins T (eds). Robbins Pathologic Basis of disease (7th edn). Philadelphia, W B Saunders, 2004; pp 269-342.

[2] Sharp L, Gould A, Harris V, et al. United Kingdom Scottish Cancer Registry 1981- 1990. In Parkin D M, Kramarova E, Drapper G J, *et al* (eds). International Incidence of Childhood Cancer (Vol 2). IARC Sci Publ No 144, Lyon, 369-371.

[3] Bunin GR, Jarreti P, Meadows AT. Greater Delaware Valley Paediatric Tumour Registry, 1970-1979: in Parkin D M, Stiller CA, Drapper GJ *et al* . (eds). International Incidence of Childhood Cancer. IARC Sci Publ No 87, Lyon, 1988, 81-86.

[4] Akang EEU. Childhood Tumours in Ibadan, Nigeria (1973-1990). Paediatric Pathology and Laboratory Medicine, 1996; 16: 791-800.

[5] Mandong BM, Angyo IA, Zoakah AI. Paediatric Solid Malignant Tumours in JUTH, Jos, (Hospital based histopathological study) Nig J Med, 2000; 9(2): 52-55.

[6] Tijani SO, Elesha SO, Bayo AA. Morpliological patterns of paediatric solid cancer in Lagos, Nigeria. West Afr J Med. 1995; 14(3): 174 – 179.

[7] Akhiwu WO, Igbe AP, Aligbe JU, Eze GI, Akang EEU. Malignant Childhood Tumours in Benin City. West Afr J Med 2009, 28(4): 222-226.

[8] Welbeck JE, Hesse AA. Pattern of childhood malignancy in Korle Bu Teaching Hospital, Ghana. West Afr. Med. J. 1998; 17(2) 81-4.

[9] Singh SK, Das D, Bhahattacharjee H, et al. A rare case of adult onset retinoblastoma. Oman J Ophthalmol 2011; 4(1): 25-27
[10] Bunin GR, Orjuela M. Geographic and environmental factors. In Singh AD, Damato BE Pe'er j, et al, eds. Clinical ophthalmic oncology. Philadelphia: Saunders-Elsevier, 2007: 410-16
[11] Parkin DM, Kramarova E, Drapper GJ et al. International incidence of childhood cancer, vol II. IARC Sci Publ 1998: 1-391
[12] Broaddus E, Topham A, Sigh AD. Incidence of retinoblastoma in the USA: 1975-2004. Br J Ophthalmol 2009; 93:21-23
[13] Pendagrass TW, Davis S. Incidence of retinoblastoma in the United States. Arch Ophthalmol 1980; 98: 1204-10
[14] MacCarthy A, Birch JM, Drapper GJ, et al. Retinoblastoma in Great Britain 1963-2002. Br J Ophthalmol 2009; 93: 33-37
[15] Seregard S, Lundell G, Svedberg H, Kivela T. Incidence of retinoblastoma from 1958 to 1998 in Northern Europe. Ophthalmol 2004;111: 1228-1232
[16] Arif M, Iqbal Z, Islam Z. Retinoblastoma in NWFP, Pakistan. J Ayub Med Coll Abbottabad 2009; 21(4): 60-62
[17] Bai S, Ren R, Shi J, et al. Retinoblastoma in the Beijing Tongren Hospital from 1957 to 2006: clinicopathological findings. Br J Ophthalmol (2010). doi:10.1136/bjo.2010.181396
[18] Freedman J, Goldberg L. Incidence of retinoblastoma in Bantu South Africa. Br J Ophthalmol 1976; 60: 655-56
[19] Kaimbo Wa Kaimbo D, Mvitu MN, Missotten L. Presenting signs of retinoblastoma in Congolese Patients. Bull Soc Belge Ophthalmol 2002; 283: 37-41
[20] Akang EE, Ajaiyeba IA, Campbell OB, Olurin IO, Aghadiuno PU. Retinoblastomas in Ibadan Nigeria-II: Clinicopathologic features. West Afr J Med 2000: 19: 6-11
[21] Chantada G, Fandino A, Manzitti J, Urutia L, Schvertzman E. Late diagnosis of retinoblastoma in a developing country. Arch Dis Child 1999; 80: 171-4
[22] Kayembe L. Retinoblastoma- 21years review. J Fr Ophthalmol 1986; 9: 651- 5
[23] Nwosu SN, Okoye GS, Ulasi TO. Delayed diagnosis of retinoblastoma. Cent Afr Med J. 1994; 40: 353-55
[24] Ben ED, Chirambo MC. Incidence of retinoblastoma in Malawi. Pediatr Ophthalmol 1976; 13: 340-43
[25] Koulibaly M, Kabba IS, Cisse A, et al. Cancer incidence in Conakry, Guinea: First results from the cancer registry 1992-1995. Int J Cancer1997; 70: 30-45
[26] Owoeye JFA, Afolayan EAO, Ademola-Popoola DS. Retinoblastoma – a clinicopathologic study in Ilorin Nigeria. Afr J Health Sci 2005; 12(3-4): 94-100
[27] Lea-Leal C, Flores-Rojo M, Medina-Samson A, et al. A multicentre report from the Mexican retinoblastoma group. Br J Ophthalmol 2004; 88: 1074-1077.
[28] Krishna SM, Yu G, Finger PT. The effect of race on retinoblastoma. J Pediatr Ophthalmol Strabismus 2009; 46 (5): 288-293.
[29] Howe HL, Wu X, Ries LA, et al. Annual report to the nation on the status of cancer, 1975-2003, featuring cancer among US Hispanic/Latino populations. Cancer 2006; 107:1711-1742

[30] Steliarova-Foucher E, Stiller C, Kaarsch P, et al. Geographical patterns and time trends of cancer incidence and survival among children and adolescents in Europe since the 1970s (the AC-CIS project): an epidemiological study. Lancet 2004; 364: 2097-2105

Part 3

Basic Sciences

6

The Retinoblastoma Family Protein p130 as a Negative Regulator of Cell Growth and Tumor Progression

Luigi Bagella[1,2]
[1]*Department of Biomedical Sciences, Division of Biochemistry and Biophysics, National Institute of Biostructures and Biosystems, University of Sassari*
[2]*Sbarro Institute for Cancer Research and Molecular Medicine, Center for Biotechnology, College of Science and Technology, Temple University, Philadelphia*
[1]*Italy*
[2]*USA*

1. Introduction

In the last years, the large amount of genomic sequences obtained after the decodification of the human genome, has made clearer the differences in the patterns of gene expression among the distinct tumor types and the equivalent normal tissues. The identification of a considerable number of differentially expressed gene products has shortened, in some measure, the bridge between correlative and causative data. Correlative genes are genes simply altered as a result of the process of transformation, and they are not responsible of critical effects upon tumor formation. In contrast, causative genes represent the basis of the malignant transformation. They play a decisive role to origin and maintain the transformed state and could be exploited for therapeutic strategies. Oncogenes and tumor suppressor genes are the most important causative genes and for this reason represent critical targets for new anticancer drug development.

Tumorigenesis proceeds through the accumulation of genetic mutations and epigenetic alterations consenting cells to break free from the tight network of controls set to regulate the homeostatic balance between cell proliferation and cell death (Baylin and Herman, 2000; Hanahan and Weinberg, 2000; Knudson, 2001; Herceg and Hainaut, 2007). The elucidation of the human genome sequence, together with the development of novel experimental techniques, has allowed the identification of genetic alterations in tumors in unprecedented details. The genetic events can be associated with the gain and loss of entire chromosomes, specific chromosomal translocations, gene amplifications, deletions or point mutations (Knudson, 1997). In addition to genetic changes, the important results obtained recently on how chromatin-remodeling enzymes controls gene transcription have underscored the crucial role of epigenetic mechanisms in the initiation and the development of cancer. Epigenetic events, such as modifications of DNA methylation patterns, and changes of chromatin structure have emerged as key mechanisms in malignant transformation (Fearon, 1997; Jones & Baylin, 2002; Baylin, 2005; Boehm & Hahn, 2011). Genetic and epigenetic events can conduct to the gain of oncogenes functions or to the loss of tumor suppressor genes (TSGs) functions, contributing to the acquired features of transformed phenotype. They represent two complementary mechanisms that are implicated in every step of carcinogenesis, from the responses to carcinogen exposures to the progression into malignancy. Autonomous cellular proliferation, immortalization, deficiencies in differentiation, induction of angiogenesis, propensity for invasion, resistance to apoptosis, induction and increased genomic instability are common characteristics of cancer cells. It has become increasingly evident that cancer is fundamentally a disease of failure of regulation of tissue growth; generally, changes in many genes are required to transform a normal cell into a cancer cell. TSGs are a family of genes that promote negative regulation on cancer cell growth inhibiting cell division and survival. Proto-oncogenes are normal genes that could become oncogenes due to mutations or to increased expression and they are able to stimulate cell proliferation and exert positive regulation of cell growth. Therefore, alterations of tumor suppressors and proto-oncogenes that may occur if the genomic integrity is compromised by intrinsic factors or exogenous agents, represent a crucial step in the transformation of a normal cell into a cancer cell (Knudson, 1985; Levine & Puzio-Kuter, 2010; Croce, 2008; Heeg, et al., 2006).

The RB1 gene represents a typical TSG, first identified in a malignant tumor of the retina known as retinoblastoma. When both the alleles of this gene are mutated, the protein (pRB) is inactivated causing the development of retinoblastoma (Knudson, 1971; Murphree & Benedict, 1984; Friend et al., 1986; Fung, et al., 1987; Lee et al., 1987a, 1987b). Retinoblastoma develops in early childhood, typically before the age of 5, and it has one of the highest cure rates of all childhood cancers, with more than 95% of patients surviving into adulthood. Retinoblastoma is a rare type of eye cancerous tumor that develops in the retina's cells. There are two forms of the disease: a heritable and a non-heritable form. In most children with retinoblastoma, the disease affects only one eye (unilateral retinoblastoma), however, one out of three children with retinoblastoma develops cancer in both eyes (bilateral retinoblastoma). Unilateral retinoblastoma represents a sporadic disease, as there is no family history for this cancer, whereas bilateral retinoblastoma represents the hereditary form and it is an autosomal dominant disease. The most common first symptom of retinoblastoma is an abnormal appearance of the pupil called "leukocoria" or "cat's eye reflex", which is a white reflection in the pupil. Other symptoms of retinoblastoma include red and irritated eyes, crossed eyes or strabismus.

In the early 1970s, Knudson postulated a model, referred to as the 'Two-hit hypothesis', with the main goal of clarifying the distinction between the two forms of retinoblastoma. A patient with inherited retinoblastoma, has a first insult already inherited in his/her own DNA, any second insult would lead to cancer, whereas a patient with non-inherited retinoblastoma, must undergo two "hits" before a tumor could develop. The identification of the retinoblastoma gene occurred in 1987 and fully confirmed Knudson's interpretation (Knudson, 1971; Lee et al., 1987a, 1987b). Indirectly, Knudson's work led to the identification of cancer-related genes and so far represents a milestone in carcinogenesis. As discussed previously, the development of cancer depends on multiple "hits" to the DNA, leading to both the activation of proto-oncogenes and the deactivation of TSGs. The activation/inactivation mechanisms of TSGs and proto-oncogenes are distinctive. Genetic changes can occur at different levels and by different mechanisms. TSGs are inactivated by "loss of function mutations" on the contrary, proto-oncogenes are activated through "gain of function mutations". In cancer cells, tumor suppressors are not functionally working and they lose the ability to control over cell proliferation. Oncogenes, instead, are constitutively activated, leading to continuous signaling which acts positively on cell growth. Unlike oncogenes, TSGs generally follow the 'two-hit hypothesis', which indicates that, before a particular outcome is manifested, both alleles of a specific gene must be affected because if only one is damaged the second can still produce the correct protein. The characteristic mechanism of this activation/inactivation phenomena means that when the cancer is promoted by the inactivation of a TSG, both the alleles of this TSG are usually inactivated whereas, when the cancer is mediated by oncogenes, the mutation of a single copy of the proto-oncogene is sufficient to activate itself, leading to cell transformation. In other words, mutant tumor suppressor's alleles are usually recessive, whereas mutant oncogene alleles are typically dominant.

pRB and the related proteins, p107 and p130, are TSGs and form the retinoblastoma (Rb) gene family. The three members of the Rb gene family have been the focus of great interest, because of their pivotal role as negative regulators of cell cycle progression. Together these proteins are also known as "pocket proteins". The term pocket protein derives from their highly conserved region, the pocket domain, which mediates interaction with viral oncoproteins as well as cellular proteins to exert the biological functions of these proteins (Graña, 1998; Cobrinik, 2005). Several examples of these interactions involving transcription factors as well as enzymes are listed in Table 1. p107 and p130 share homologies throughout the entire length of the protein, whereas their homology with pRB is limited to the conserved A and B domains. The genes are located on different chromosomes and the expression of the proteins is differently regulated throughout the cell cycle (Lee et al., 1987a; Hong et al., 1989; Yeung et al., 1993; Mayol et al., 1993; Paggi et al., 1996; Ichimura et al., 2000). They interact with different E2F proteins, thereby blocking different subsets of gene promoters, but have in common that this interaction is regulated through phosphorylation by cyclin-dependent kinases (cdks) (Hurford et al., 1997; Classon et al., 2000; Stiegler & Giordano, 2001; Sun, 2007). In fact, all the Rb family members exert their function interfering, between the others, with the coordinated regulation of the enzymatic activity of cdks, which are key regulatory factors of the cell cycle progression (Graña & Reddy, 1995; Morgan, 1995 & 1997). The cdks and their heterodimeric cyclin partners represents prime targets for the development of new inhibitors and anticancer therapeutic strategies. During the last decades, several chemical compounds with remarkable cdk inhibitory activity have been described. These molecules are starting to become a significant therapeutic asset in the treatment of cancer. Among the small molecules, peptides, with a comparable cdk inhibitory activity, are emerging as a novel class of drugs for cancer therapy. Cdk2 is considered the prototypic cell cycle kinase. It represents an excellent runner in the development of anticancer therapeutics not only because of its crucial role to pass through the G1 restriction checkpoint and to drive cells into DNA replication but also because its alteration is a pathogenic hallmark of tumorigenesis (McDonald & El-Deiry, 2000; Fischer, 2004; Whittaker et al., 2004; Dai & Grant, 2004; Shapiro, 2006; de Cárcer et al., 2007; Malumbres & Barbacid, 2009; Cirillo, et al., 2011). p130 together with p107 has the ability to inhibit the kinase activity

Rb family protein	Protein partner	Biological function of the protein partner	Biological role of the Rb family protein
pRB	Cyclin D	CDK subunit	Cell cycle
	E2Fs	Transcription factors	Cell cycle
	c-Jun	Transcription factor	Cell cycle
	c-Myc	Transcription factor	Cell cycle
	Spl	Transcription factor	Cell cycle
	Abl	Nuclear tyrosine kinase	Cell cycle
	Che-1	Transcription factor	Cell cycle
	Id-2	Transcription factor-corepressor	Cell cycle
	MCM7	DNA replication licensing factor	Inhibition of DNA replication
	RBAp48	Histone deacetylase complex factor	Growth inhibition
	TAFII250/TFII D	Transcription factor	Transcription
	HDAC1	Histone deacetylase	Transcription
	BRG1	Transcription factor	Transcription
	MyoD	Transcription factor	Muscle differentiation
	HBP1	Transcription factor	Muscle differentiation
	p202	Transcription factor	Muscle differentiation
	NF-IL6	Transcription factor	Adipocyte differentiation
p130	Cyclins A and E	CDK subunits	Cell cycle
	E2Fs	Transcription factors	Cell cycle
	MCM7	DNA replication licensing factor	Inhibition of DNA replication
	HDAC1	Histone deacetylase	Transcription
	HBP1	Transcription factor	Muscle differentiation
p107	Cyclins A and E	CDK subunits	Cell cycle
	E2Fs	Transcription factors	Cell cycle
	c-Myc	Transcription factor	Cell cycle
	Spl	Transcription factor	Cell cycle
	MCM7	DNA replication licensing factor	Inhibition of DNA replication
	HDAC1	Histone deacetylase	Transcription
	MyoD	Transcription factor	Muscle differentiation

Table 1. The biological roles of the Rb family proteins are mainly dependent on their ability to interact and modulate the activities of cellular proteins

of the cdk2/cyclins A and cdk2/cyclins E complexes (Adams, 1996; Woo, 1997; Lacy, 1997; De Luca, 1997). Specifically, p107 is able to inhibit their kinase activity recruiting or mimicking a cyclin-dependent kinase inhibitor (CKI) p21 (Zhu et al., 1995; Adams, 1996). Whereas, p130 is able to physically bind to the Cdk2/Cyclins A and Cdk2/Cyclin E complexes suggesting that part of its growth suppressor function could be mediated by the inhibition of this essential cell cycle kinase. The inhibitory activity of p130 has been attributed to the spacer region (De Luca, 1997). Recently, a 39 amino acid long p130 spacer-derived peptide termed "Spa310" has been identified as responsible of the cdk2-dependent kinase inhibitory activity proving to be an excellent candidate in a mechanism-based approach in cancer therapy (Bagella, 2007; Giordano, 2007a, 2007b).

2. p130, Rb family proteins and LXCXE-like motif

The p130 protein, together with p105 and p107, is a member of the Rb family of tumor suppressors. The three members of this family share high degree of homology and biological functions (Lee et al., 1987a; Ewen et al., 1991; Mayol et al., 1993; Li et al., 1993; Paggi et al., 1996; Mayol & Graña, 1997; Nevins, 1998). All of them are characterized by two highly conserved functional domains termed A and B, which are separated by a spacer region, which differs between all the three Rb family members. They are also called "pocket proteins" because the two domains, A and B, are assembled into a pocket-like structure for the presence of the spacer region (figure 1) (Graña, 1998; Cobrinik, 2005; Du & Pogoriler, 2006; Macaluso et al., 2006; Sun et al., 2007). The pocket domain sequence of all the three pocket members is well known for its ability to interact with proteins containing LXCXE motifs (Lee et al., 1998; Dahiya et al., 2000). The LXCXE domain is composed by a small block of highly conserved amino-acid residues counting the sequence leucine-X-cysteine-X-glutamate, where the letter 'X' indicates any amino acids. A large selection of proteins containing an LXCXE-like sequence is able to interact with the Rb family proteins.

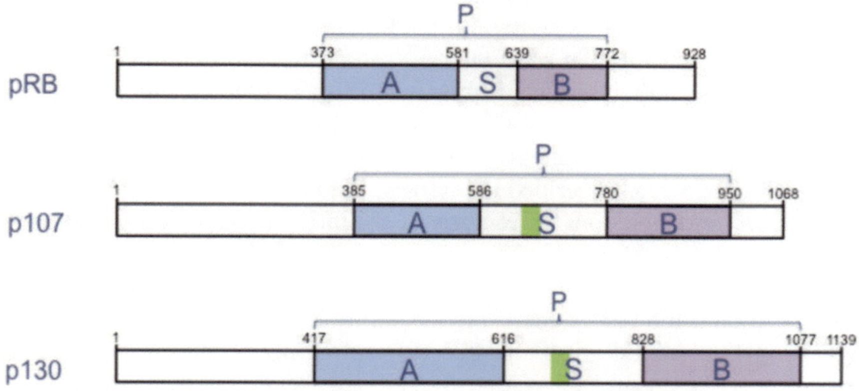

Fig. 1. Schematic diagram of the amino acid sequences of the retinoblastoma family proteins highlighting the relative locations of functional domains within each member (N-terminus to the right, C-terminus to the left). The retinoblastoma family consists of pRb, p107 and p130. P indicates the pocket domain, responsible for most protein–protein interactions, composed by two conserved domains A and B, separated by the spacer region S. The green box specifies the conserved sequence motif, between p107 and p130, responsible for binding the Cdk/Cyclin complexes.

The DNA virus oncoprotein, E1A (the early-region 1A of the human adenovirus type 5), was identified by coimmunoprecipitation with pRB. E1A contains an LXCXE motif that is responsible for this interaction (Whyte, et al. 1989; Nielsch et al., 1991; Rumpf et al., 1999). The pRB pocket domain has been co-crystallized with an LXCXE peptide, allowing localization of the LXCXE binding site on the inside of its B domain sequence (Lee et al., 1998). Also, the other members of the Rb family, p107 and p130, are able to bind E1A through a similar mechanism (Herrmann et al., 1991; Putzer et al., 1997; Lee et al., 2002; Xiao et al., 2003). Together with adenovirus E1A, other DNA virus oncoproteins such as human papillomavirus (HPV) E7 and Simian virus 40 large T antigen, contain LXCXE-like sequences which are used to bind to the Rb family proteins inhibiting their functions and promoting cell transformation and consequently cancer development (Hu et al., 1990; Ciccolini et al., 1994; Jones et al. 1997; Dahiya et al., 2000; Caldeira et al. 2000; Münger et al., 2001; Helt & Galloway, 2003; Caracciolo et al., 2006; Felsani et al., 2006). Moreover, an LXCXE-like motif was also found in several cellular proteins such as, histone deacetylases 1 and 2 (HDAC1 and HDAC2), protein phosphatase 1 (PP1), breast cancer type 1 (BRCA1), and Brahma-Related Gene 1 (BRG1), interacting with Rb family proteins, are involved in their pathways and play important roles for their functions. (Dunaief et al., 1994; Fan et al., 2001; Rayman et al., 2002; Dunaief et al., 2002). The Rb family proteins are essential regulators of the cell cycle. They play a crucial role during the cell cycle, primarily through their ability to bind members of the E2F family and to block the activation of genes involved in cell cycle progression (Moberg et al., 1996; Sidle et al., 1996; Stiegler & Giordano, 1999; Macaluso et al., 2006; Sun et al., 2007). The E2F family members play a major role during the G1/S cell cycle transition. Based on their functions they can be divided in two distinctive groups: transcription activators and repressors (figure 2). The E2F(1-3a) members are activators and promote and help carry out the cell cycle, while the E2F(3b-8) factors are repressors and inhibit the cell cycle. The E2F(1-6) proteins bind to DNA as heterodimers, in association with the dimerization partner DP1 or DP2, increasing the E2F binding stability (Johnson et al., 1993; Zheng et al., 1999; Gaubatz et al., 2000; Cobrinik, 2005; Chen et al., 2009). Although the E2F factors are able to bind the Rb family proteins, they do not possess any LXCXE domains, suggesting that most of them should have a different pocket protein-binding domain. This observation was confirmed in studies focused on mutational analysis. In these studies, the mutation of the LXCXE binding site did not prevent pRB from binding and inactivating the E2F factors, whereas, these mutations inhibited the interactions with HDAC1 and HDAC2. Indeed, as described previously, both HDAC1 and HDAC2 contain an LXCXE-like sequence, and deletions of regions of the proteins containing this sequence preclude their binding to pocket proteins (Dunaief et al., 1994; Magnaghi-Jaulin et al., 1998; Ferreira et al., 1998; Fan et al., 2001). Thus, the LXCXE binding site mutations consent to distinct the ability to bind the E2F factors from the ability to efficiently recruit HDAC1 and HDAC2, suggesting that inhibition of the E2F activity alone is not sufficient to sustain actively repress transcription and consequently cell growth arrest (Dahiya et al., 2000). Therefore, it would seem that effective growth suppression by pocket proteins requires not only the interaction with the E2F factors, but also the recruitment of HDAC1 and HDAC2, providing evidence that the LXCXE binding site is important for their efficient function. Further studies underscored that other chromatin remodeling enzymes such as BRG1 and Brahma (BRM), that are components of the human SWI–SNF nucleosome-remodeling complex, are able to cooperate with the pocket protein-related cell growth suppression (Dunaief et al., 1994; Ferreira et al., 1998; Brehm et al. 1998; Ross et al., 1999; Zhang et al.,

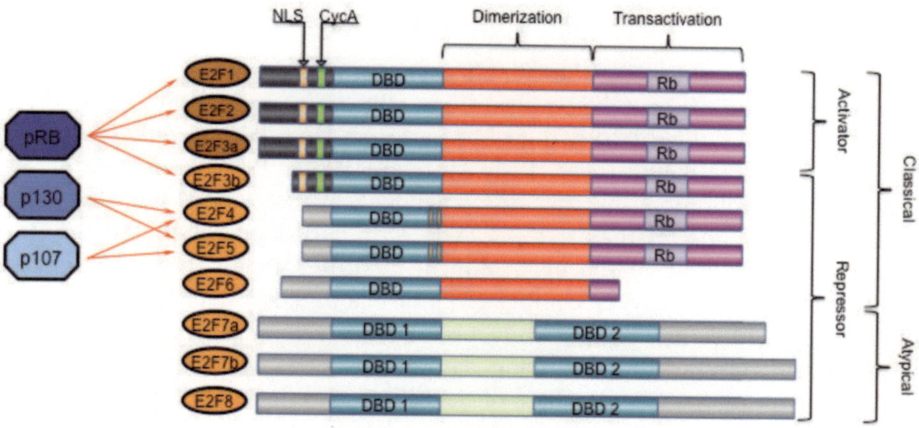

Fig. 2. Structural organization of E2F transcription factors and their interactions with Rb family proteins. E2Fs can be subdivided into activator factors: E2F1, E2F2, E2F3a and repressor factors: E2F3b, E2F4, E2F5, E2F6, E2F7a, E2F7b and E2F8. They can also be divided in Classical and Atypical E2Fs. The most peculiar differences between Classical E2Fs, and Atypical E2Fs are shown: Classical E2Fs (E2F1-6), bind to DNA only after coupling with a second protein, called dimerization partner protein (DP). Through their dimerization domain, they form heterodimers with DP1 and DP2 proteins to allow the binding to DNA. Atypical E2Fs, E2F(7-8), show a duplicated DNA binding domain (DBD) that allow to bind to DNA in a DP-independent manner (as a homodimer). For a review about this class of E2F proteins see: Lammens et al., 2009. The classical E2Fs have also a transactivation domain that contains the Rb family proteins binding motif (Rb). pRB preferentially binds to the activator factors E2F1, E2F2, and E2F3a and the repressor factor E2F3b. p107 and p130 preferentially bind to the repressor factors E2F4 and E2F5. E2F(6-8) do not bind to pocket proteins. NLS and CycA indicate the nuclear localization signal and the Cyclin A binding motif respectively.

2000; Kadam & Emerson, 2003). Several reports showed that active repression mediated by p130 and pRB could involve a molecular mechanism by which condensed chromatin structure is enhanced not only through histone deacetylation but also through methylation. Macaluso and colleagues proposed multimolecular complexes bound to the estrogen receptor-α (ER-α) in breast cancer containing the histone methyl transferase (SUV39H1) and the DNA-(cytosine-5) methyltransferase 1 (*DNMT1)* together with p130-E2F4(5) and HDAC1 suggesting a novel link between p130 and chromatin-modifying enzymes in the transcriptional regulation of the ER-α gene.

In addition, other studies demonstrated that Polycomb group (PcG) proteins, another class of remodel chromatin proteins, interact with Rb family proteins and that these associations are important links between the transcriptional repression activities related to the pocket proteins and polycomb pathways (Dahiya et al. 2001; Bracken et al. 2003; Kotake et al., 2007; Tonini et al., 2004 & 2008). Although the large number of observations underline how the transcriptional repression's mechanisms of the Rb family members have been extensively investigated, so far the contribution of the chromatin remodeling enzymes and pocket proteins to physically repress responsive promoters in G0 and early G1 is still debated, and represents an important unresolved piece of this issue.

3. p130, hypho/hyperphoshorilation and regulation of E2F-responsive genes

One key mechanism controlling the G0/G1 checkpoint is the phosphorylation of the Rb family proteins by the cdk/cyclin complexes. The cdks are serine and threonine kinases and encompass a family divided into two groups based on their roles in cell cycle progression and transcriptional regulation (Lees, 1995; Morgan, 1995 & 1997; Napolitano et al., 2002; Shapiro, 2006). By definition, the cdks are dependent on associations with their activating subunits, termed cyclins for their cyclical expression and degradation. All the Rb family proteins contain several serine or threonine residues that can be recognized and phosphorylated by the cdk/cyclin complexes (Sidle et al., 1996; Mayol & Grana, 1998). In the hypophosphorylated state, the Rb family proteins are active and carry out their role as tumor suppressors binding and inhibiting, as previously described, transcription factors of the E2F family during the G0/G1 phase of the cell cycle. When it is time for a cell to enter the S phase, the cdk/cyclin complexes phosphorylate the pocket proteins, inhibiting their activity. For instance, increased phosphorylation of pRB decreases the affinity to E2F1 that dissociate from the pocket protein and becomes active allowing the progression of the cell cycle. The phosphorylation state of p130 occurs in all the mechanisms of growth regulation associated with this protein, this event is obviously cell cycle regulated as p130 has been shown to be a substrate for the cdk/cyclin complexes (Baldi et al., 1995; Canhoto et al., 2000; Hansen et al., 2001). In comparison to the other Rb family members, the p130 expression levels change during the cell cycle; in fact p130 is the most abundant in the G0 phase (Kiess et al., 1995) and differs from the others also in its phosphorylated status. Indeed, it has been described that p130 undergoes phosphorylation at distinctive sites during the G0 phase in a way that characterizes p130 from the other members of the Rb family proteins (Kiess et al., 1995; Canhoto et al., 2000). p130 is phosphorylated by the Cdk4/Cyclin D or Cdk6/Cyclin D and Cdk2/Cyclin E or Cdk2/Cyclin A complexes and its expression levels fall when the cells enter into the S phase (Baldi et al., 1995; Mayol et al., 1995; Claudio et al., 1996; Dong et al., 1998; Tedesco et al., 2002). *In vivo* phosphorylation mapping of human p130 identified 22 serine and threonine residues, targeted by the kinases Cdk2, Cdk4 and Cdk6 (Hansen et al., 2001). These residues can be divided into four groups. The first group is positioned between the end of the N-terminal region and the beginning of the A domain. It consists of three residues; one is common to all the three Rb family members, one is shared with p107, and the last one is unique to p130. The second group contains six residues that are located in the spacer region; three out of six are unique to p130, the rest are common to p107. The third group is located within the B domain and contains seven residues; six out of seven are unique to p130, one is shared with p107. Finally, the last group is situated in the C-terminal region and contains six residues; two are common to all the three proteins, two are shared with p107 and the remaining two are unique to p130. In total, three out of 22 residues share homology with all the three Rb family members; ten are common to p107, while, twelve are apparently unique to p130 (figure 3). The carboxy-terminal region of p130 is important in coordinating the function of the whole protein. The C-terminus differs in length and similarity to the one of pRB, while it is very comparable to the p107's, considering that, as already extensively mentioned, they are more strictly related to each other. Indeed, the C-terminus of p130 and p107 contains in addition to HADC-1 (Stiegler et al., 1998) and cdk/cyclin complex binding domain (Hansen et al., 2001), independent nuclear localization signals (NLS) that could target reporter proteins to the nucleus (Chestukhin et al., 2002). Hypophosphorylated p130 interacts with the E2F4, and E2F5 transcriptional factors, forming

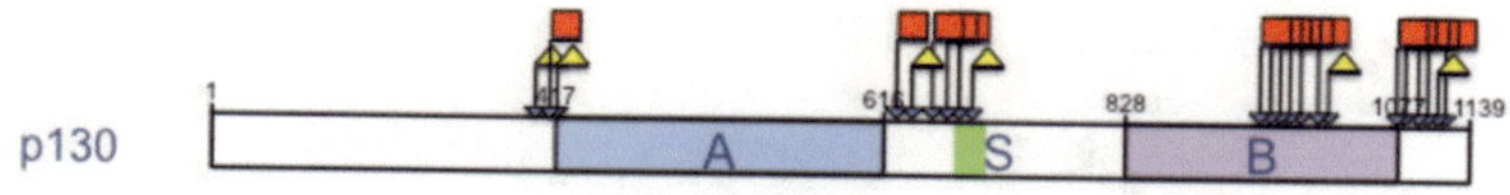

Fig. 3. Schematic summary of the 22 serine or threonine amino acids, identified by in vivo phosphorylation assays of p130, which are targets for Cdk2/Cyclin A(B) and Cdk4(6)/Cyclin D. A, B and S refer to p130 domains. The red square and the yellow triangle indicate the serine and the threonine residues respectively.

the p130/E2F4(5) repressor complexes. E2F4 and E2F5 are considered poor transcriptional activators due, in part, to their lack of a NLS. The dependence of cellular localization of these E2F transcription factors suggests that p130 may be involved in nucleocytoplasmic trafficking. An accumulation of the p130/E2F4(5) complexes have been shown when cells are quiescent or differentiating, whereas the ability of p130 to bind E2F4(5) is inhibited when cells are entering late G1/S phase of the cell cycle suggesting that the involvement of these complexes is critical during the G0/G1 phase (Dimova and Dyson, 2005). Indeed, E2F4 and E2F5 are expressed throughout the cell cycle, but they are more present in G0/G1 phase, when they can be associated and recruited to the nucleus by p130 in order to form transcriptional repressor complexes (Chestukhin et al., 2002). The p130/E2F4(5) complexes exert their repressive action recruiting to their promoters binding site, the chromatin modulating factors HDAC1, resulting in the removal of acetyl groups from the histones H3 and H4 and generating a compacted chromatin structure that is refractory to the transcription initiation (Smith et al., 1996; Iavarone & Massague, 1999; Takahashi et al., 2000; Ferreira et al., 1998 & 2001; Rayman et al., 2002). A schematic representation of the repressive action of the p130/E2F4(5) complexes is illustrated in figure 4. As showed by several scientific publications, the largest part of the E2F-responsive promoters bound E2F-4 and p130 or in alternative p107, whereas only a limited set of promoters show evidently, an interaction of the pRB/E2F(1-3) complexes (Liu et al., 2005).

In addition, it has been demonstrated that these interactions occur at very low concentration levels (Wells et al., 2000; Takahashi et al., 2000; Morrison et al., 2002; Rayman et al., 2002). Among these, the binding of pRB/E2F(1-3) to the E2F-responsive promoter of Cyclin E represent an important example (Hurford et al., 1997; Le Cam et al., 1999; Polanowska et al., 2001).

As previously indicated, the Cdk4(6)/Cyclin D and Cdk2/cyclin E(A) complexes have been involved in the phosphorylation of all the Rb family proteins (Weinberg, 1995). Although phosphorylation of the Rb family members is very often overturned by dephosphorylation, in particular circumstances, phosphorylation leads to a non-reversible inactivation. Phosphorylation of p130 starts most probably through its C-terminus and leads to the release of HDAC1 binding to the protein (Stiegler et al., 1998; Harbour et al., 1999). The following hyperphosphorylation displaces E2F4(5) from the p130 repressor complexes, leading to the release of the E2F4(5) transcription factors from p130. Unbound E2F4(5) can now migrate to the cytoplasm, while the E2F(1-3) factors are able to bind and activate their responsive promoters. It has been shown that in certain conditions, the E2F(1-3) factors bind to different promoter regions from those made vacant by E2F4(5) (Araki et al., 2003; Zhu et al., 2004). For many promoters, the binding of E2F(1-3) restore histone acetylation by the recruitment of histone acetyltransferases (HATs), which produce a more relaxed chromatin

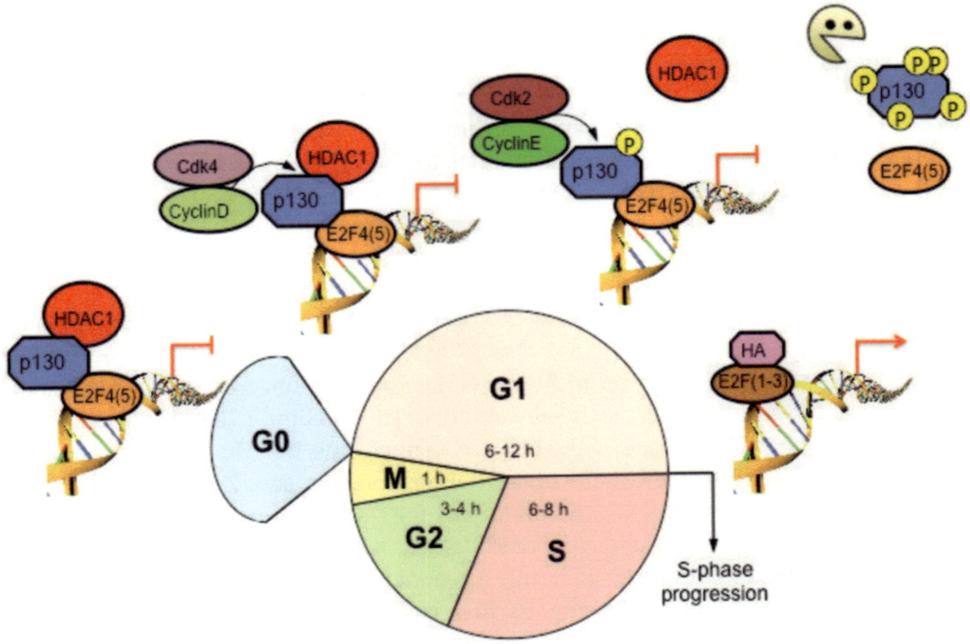

Fig. 4. A simplified view of p130/E2F4(5) complexes at E2F-responsive promoters. For simplicity several cofactors of the complexes (DP proteins or chromatin modifying enzyme) have been ignored. During G0 and early G1, p130 in complex with E2F4(5) is located at E2F-responsive promoters and exert its repressive action recruiting the chromatin modulating factors HDAC1. Phosphorylation of p130 leads to the disruption of the complexes, and E2F-responsive promoters can be activated by E2F(1-3)/HA. Hyperphosphorylated p130 can be degraded through the ubiquitin proteasomal pathway. For more detailed explanations return to text.

state that makes it accessible directly to the transcription factors and allows the cells to proliferate (Ferreira et al., 1998; Takahashi et al., 2000; Taubert et al., 2004). The hyperphosphorylation of p130 leads to its degradation through the ubiquitin proteasomal pathway (Ludlow et al., 1993; Mayol & Grana, 1997 & 1998; Smith et al., 1998; Vuocolo et al., 2003). The ubiquitination of p130 is followed by proteasomal degradation in late G1, which rapidly decreases the expression level of the protein when cells enter in S phase (Tedesco et al., 2002). Thus, p130 is removed when the cells are stimulated to enter a proliferative status confirming that its main relevant function is to arrest cells to G0 phase and to sustain them in this phase when the cells are in a quiescent status or begin to differentiate.

4. p130, cell growth arrest and tumor suppression

One of the most important key factors involved in the origin of a malignant cellular phenotype is the TSGs inactivation. As previously discussed, pRB, p107 and p130, in addition to their similar structural characteristics, share parallel biological functions. The abilities of inhibiting E2F-responsive promoters, recruiting chromatin-remodeling enzymes and actively repressing transcription (Classon & Dyson, 2001; Burkhart & Sage, 2008) confirms that these proteins show extensive overlapping functions and compensatory effects at cell cycle level. Indeed, fibroblasts lacking one of the three pocket proteins are still able to sustain growth arrest in G0/G1 phase, but, on the other hand, fibroblasts lacking all of the three Rb family proteins lose this biological function (Sage et al., 2000; Dannenberg et al., 2000). Notwithstanding all the Rb family proteins show redundant actions *in vitro*, they clearly have distinct functions in a number of cell types *in vivo*. pRB-deficient mice die during the period of middle gestation showing a large number of anomalies in neural and hematopoietic development, however, $p107^{-/-}$ and $p130^{-/-}$ mice show neonatal lethality with reduced limb and defective chondrocyte growth and endochondral ossification (Clarke et al., 1992; Cobrinik et al., 1996). Given that p107/p130-deficient mice have a normal development during gestation in comparison to $RB^{-/-}$ mice, is reasonable to believe that pocket protein functions cannot be considered completely compensatory (Zhu et al., 1993; Claudio et al., 1994). In addition, other studies highlight elevated proliferation, apoptosis and defective differentiation in liver, brain, muscle, eye, skin, and placenta of pRB-deficient mouse embryos (Liu et al., 2004), whereas p130-/p107-deficient mouse embryos display defects in a different and limited set of tissues (Ruiz et al., 2003; Vanderluit et al., 2004). Although it is possible to speculate with all the statements considered so far, the main reason why the three pocket proteins show redundant effect in some cases whereas, in other cases they lose these compensatory functions is poorly understood. Certainly, given the large spectrum of cells and tissue that have been analyzed, it cannot be excluded that these compensatory effects are more often cell type dependent, but, on the other hand, since p130 owns strict similarity with p107 both in structure and biological functions, it is reasonable to consider that p130 shows a major compensatory effect with p107 in comparison to pRB. For instance, p130-deficient T lymphocytes exhibit normal proliferation *in vitro* and normal cell-mediated immune function *in vivo*, but they show high levels of p107, which is able to replace p130 interacting with E2F4(5) and to form p107/E2F4(5) repressor complexes (Mulligan et al., 1998). Instead, a recent finding demonstrates that p107 and p130 have distinct biological functions to regulate pulmonary epithelial proliferation and survival. In murine models with conditional pocket proteins-deficient lung epithelium, p107 cooperates with pRB to suppress proliferation, however, p130, not being involved in cell growth arrest, exerts a pro-apoptotic function (Simpson et al., 2009). These clinical investigations confirm, as just described above, that although the three proteins share many structural features and are able to work as negative regulators of cell proliferation, they are not temporally and functionally redundant. The inactivation of p130 function can be owed by genetic or epigenetic mechanisms or by the interaction with viral oncoproteins. Numerous melanomas for instance, contain deletion in the chromosomal region (16q12.2) where p130 gene is encoded (Yeung et al., 1993). It has been demonstrated by numerous studies that ectopic expression of human p130 in many human cancer cell lines led to a cell cycle arrest in G1 phase of the cell cycle. For instance, the overexpression of p130 is able to arrest in G1 phase the human T98G glioblastoma cell line, whereas the same cell line does not respond with a G1 arrest after overexpression of the other two members of the Rb family (Claudio et al., 1994). This result is further evidence that the biological functions of the three Rb family proteins are not totally compensatory. The nasopharyngeal HONE-1, cell line displays a strong reduction in the expression level of p130, suggesting a possible involvement of this protein in nasopharyngeal carcinogenesis. Constitutive expression of p130 causes a considerable reduction in HONE-1 cell proliferation and significant changes in cellular morphology (Claudio et al., 1994; Claudio et al., 2000a).

Furthermore, retrovirus-mediated delivery of wild-type p130 shows growth arrest and tumor progression reduction in a lung tumor cell line, H23, and in xeno-transplanted nude mice respectively (Claudio et al., 2000b). The p130 tumor suppressor gene is functionally inactivated in a broad range of cancers. Inactivation of its biological function has been described in different gynecological malignancies. Frequent loss of heterozygosity (LOH) to chromosome 16q12.2, where p130 maps, have been described in ovarian cancer. A large study on ovarian carcinomas displays a drop of the expression level of p130 by 40% and this result correlates inversely with tumor grade (D'Andrilli et al., 2004). In breast cancer, a similar study highlights a reduction of p130 expression level, more recurrent in lobular than in ductal carcinomas, which significantly correlates with estrogen receptor and progesterone receptor-B (Milde-Langosch et al., 2001). Furthermore, p130, in a complex with chromatin-modifying enzymes, takes part in the transcriptional regulation of the ER-α modifying histone acetylation and DNA methylation pattern (Macaluso et al., 2003). A p130 involvement has been also suggested in lung tumor. Low expression level of p130 has been reported in small cell lung cancer (SCLC) and this result inversely correlates with histologic grade, proliferation, and patient survival (Baldi et al., 1996; Helin et al., 1997; Caputi et al., 2002; Cinti et al., 2005). An explanation of p130 deregulation in lung cancer has been recently proposed. CTCF, a chromatin insulator CCCTC-binding factor, is involved in the transcriptional activity of p130 in lung fibroblasts, whereas, in lung cancer cells, a paralog of CTCF, BORIS, impairs the activity of CTCF to control p130 gene transcription (Fiorentino et al., 2011). Furthermore, a conditional triple-knockout murine model able to remove p130, pRB, and p53 in lung epithelial cells, pointed out that loss of p130 leads to a significant increment of cell proliferation and small cell lung cancer (SCLC) development (Schaffer et al., 2010). A deregulation of the p130 biological function has been shown in numerous hematological malignancies. For instance, in AIDS-related non-Hodgkin's lymphomas, an unusual high expression level of p130 has been detected, and, it was found interacting with the HIV-1 Tat protein resulting in deregulation of its tumor suppressor function (Lazzi et al., 2002). Mutations of p130 gene, involving the putative NLS, have been detected in Burkitt's lymphoma cell lines and primary tumors (Cinti et al., 2000). Interestingly, ectopic expression of p130 in the same cell lines recovers growth control (De Falco et al., 2007). Inactivation of the biological function of p130 has also been described in other malignant transformation, such as mesothelioma (Mutti et al., 1998), and nasopharyngeal carcinomas (NPC) (Claudio et al., 1994; Claudio et al., 2000a). Furthermore, an involvement of p130 has been also suggested in retinoblastoma (Bellan et al., 2002).

5. p130, Cdk2 inhibition and Spa310

As extensively previously described the mammalian cell cycle requires the coordinated expression of a family of serine/threonine protein kinases (cdks) that are activated at specific points of the cell cycle by the interaction with their regulatory subunits, cyclins (Graña & Reddy, 1995; Morgan, 1995 & 1997). The active cdk/cyclin complexes phosphorylate target proteins on cdk consensus sites, resulting in changes of their structure that are physiologically crucial for cell cycle progression. Alongside the cdk/cyclin complexes, a family of proteins that exerts cdk inhibitory activity is vital for cell cycle regulation. These proteins called cyclin-dependent kinases inhibitors (CKI) bind to the cdk alone or to the cdk/cyclin complex and regulate the cdk activity. This class of proteins consists of two groups: the INK4 and Cip/Kip proteins. The INK4 members include p15, p16, p18, p19, which specifically inactivate Cdk4 and Cdk6. They form stable complexes with the two kinases alone before their association with cyclin D (Cánepa, et al., 2007). The second class of inhibitors, the Cip/Kip proteins, includes p21, p27 and p57. Their inhibitory actions occur through the interaction and inactivation of all the G1-cdk/cyclin complexes (Besson et al., 2008). In summary, these CKIs can indirectly inhibit the E2F-mediated transcription through the interaction and inhibition of cdk/cyclin complexes that, maintaining the Rb family proteins in a hypophosphorylated state, allow them to sequester the E2F transcription factors (figure 5). Notwithstanding the wide variety of functions of the pocket proteins is E2F-responsive genes dependent, p130, as well as p107, is able to suppress cell growth through its interaction with two significant cell cycle complexes mentioned

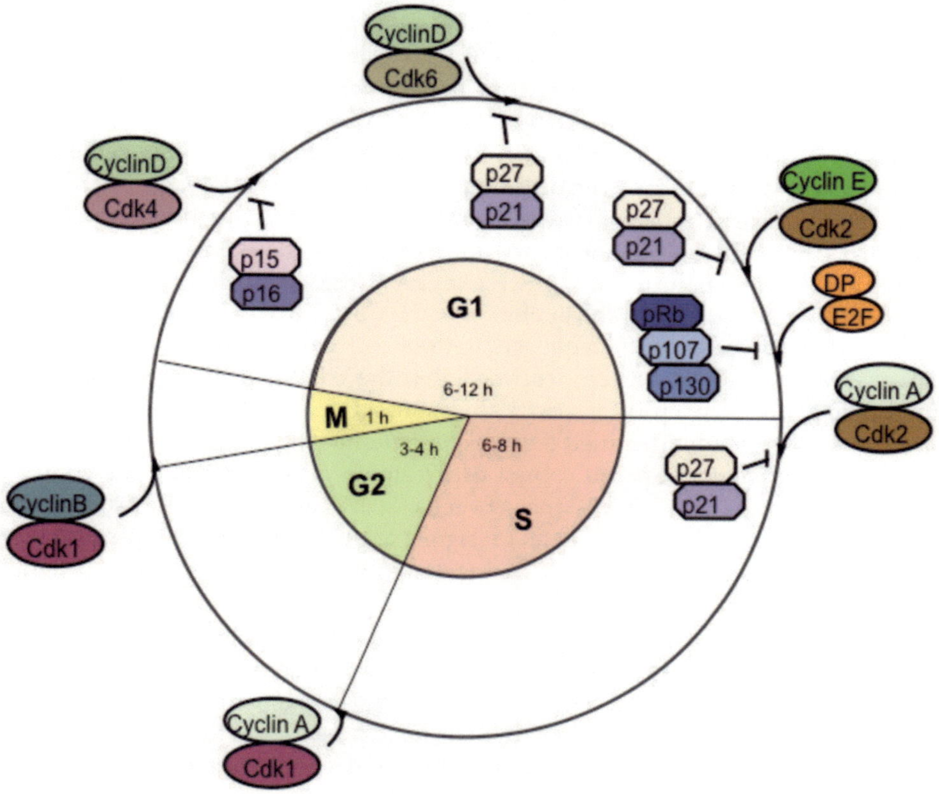

Fig. 5. A schematic representation of the main cdk/cyclin complexes involved in cell cycle control. The passage through the four phases of the cell cycle is regulated by the activities of cdks controlled by the synthesis of the appropriate cyclins during a specific phase of the cell cycle. Cell cycle inhibitory proteins, called cyclin-dependent kinase Inhibitors (CKI), can counteract cdk activity. P15, p16, p21 and p27 represent the main CKIs that specifically prevent accumulated G1-Cdk/Cyclins from acting. The G1-Cdk/Cyclin complexes [(Cdk4(6)/Cyclin D and Cdk2/Cyclin E(A)] control the G1/S checkpoint by the phosphorylation of a variety of proteins. The Rb family proteins represent one key target. Their phosphorylation prevents the binding and inactivation of the E2F transcription factors. The activation of E2Fs allows the transcription of various gene products that are indispensable to trigger S phase.

above, Cdk2/Cyclin A and Cdk2/Cyclin E (Zhu et al., 1995; Lacy & Whyte, 1997). To date, only p130 and p107 are able to bind and inhibit Cdk2/Cyclin A and Cdk2/Cyclin E through independent E2F mechanisms. Certainty, Cyclin E expression is essentially regulated by pRB, as results in pRB deficient cells where Cyclin E levels increase with the parallel disappearance of this protein, but, as mentioned previously, the role of pRB in the regulation of cyclin E occurs through crucial E2F-responsive genes (Le Cam et al., 1999; Polanowska et al., 2001). Inhibition of Cdk2/Cyclin A(E) activity by p130 underlines the fundamental role of p130 during the cell cycle, which is not only the maintenance of a G0 arrest in quiescent or differentiated cells, but also the fact that this protein can exert a control during the transition from G1- to S-phase. This inhibition halts the cells in G1 phase preventing their passing beyond the restriction point G1/S. In order for the cells to progress through G1 phase, p130 as well as all the other related proteins p107 and pRB must be phosphorylated and therefore inactivated by Cdk2/Cyclin A(E) (also by Cdk4(6)/Cyclin D). In this regard, repression of this enzymatic kinase activity by p130 might represent a decisive step to inhibit progression into S-phase. This inhibition can be considered similar to the one performed by the CKI family, and, in certain situations, can work redundantly in support of these proteins. It has been also shown that in p27-/- fibroblasts, an inhibition of Cck2 activity occurs after interaction with p130, which prevents S phase entry. This result confirms that p130, although is not related to the CKI p27, takes its place for the cyclin-dependent kinase inhibition, restoring physiologically cdk regulation (Coats et al., 1999). Moreover, it is hypothesized that the inhibition of the Cdk2 activity by p130 is the result of a direct interaction between specific sequences in the structural domains of this protein and of the kinase. Previously, it has been described that the cdk2-dependent kinase inhibitory activity shown by the pRb2/p130 is specifically confined to the p130 spacer region (De Luca et al., 1997). A recent study identified a polypeptide termed Spa310, which is mainly based on the p130 spacer region. Spa310 consist of 39 amino acids, spanning the p130 spacer region between the 641 and 679 residues (Bagella, 2007; Giordano, 2007a, 2007b). *In vitro* studies confirmed that Spa310 is able to significantly inhibit cdk2-dependent histone phosphorylation. In addition, its ectopic expression in mouse fibroblast shows a significant arrest of proliferation in the G_0/G_1 phase of the cell cycle. Interestingly, the small peptide Spa310 completely maintains the ability, typical of the full-length spacer region of p130, to inhibit cdk2 kinase activity and equally, when introduced into cells, induces growth arrest and inhibits the endogenous cdk2 activity, in an analogous manner to the spacer domain. In addition, Spa310 is also able to reduce human lung tumor growth in xeno-transplanted nude mice suggesting its potential role as a promising new type of mechanism-based drug for the treatment of malignant disorders. This therapeutic approach is focus of great interest in cancer therapy and consequently, pharmacological compounds, like small molecules, or peptides such as Spa310, targeting certain cdks, are potential points of intervention for drug discovery, since they could create rationally designed inhibitors of particular pathways that lead to malignant transformation. Over the last decade, a variety of pharmacological compounds with potent cdk inhibitory and strong anti-tumor activities have been identified and, for some of them, their potential anticancer function has been confirmed in preclinical studies (Dai & Grant, 2004; Shapiro, 2006; de Cárcer et al., 2007; Malumbres & Barbacid, 2009). The development of biological molecules, rather than chemical compounds, represent a larger line of research, since combines the efficacy of arresting cellular proliferation by interacting specifically with peculiar regulators of the cell cycle. The specificity of these compounds, compared to the non-specificity of chemical compounds, would allow the development of new molecules with better pharmacodynamics, higher patient tolerability and fewer side effects.

6. Conclusions

As broadly discussed in this chapter, a breakdown of the cell cycle caused by an unbalanced perturbation that pushes a cell to stimulate its own growth, resisting to inhibitory signals that might otherwise stop its growth, represents a common hallmark of the malignant transformation and tumor development. The assortment of all the observations here described, taken together with the further evidences available in the large body of literature, supports the scientific relevance of the p130 biological functions in cell cycle control, in cell transformation, and tumor formation.

The development of small molecules with cdk inhibitory activity, as well as the small peptides mimicking, as discussed here, the functional motifs of p130 and the preservation of its cyclin-dependent kinase inhibition, represent key tools to clarify the connections among cdks and TSGs with cell cycle progression and malignant transformation. Meanwhile, additional studies that might elucidate how the loss of function of p130, and the related pocket proteins pRB and p107, merges with the activation or the inactivation of other gene products to develop retinoblastoma or other proliferative disorders, will open up novel horizons for the biology of cancer, which will hopefully lead to the development of innovative pharmacological approaches and efficient therapies.

7. Acknowledgments

This work was supported by grants from "*Fondazione Banco di Sardegna*". I am grateful to Valeria Giola for her editorial assistance.

8. References

Adams, P.D., Sellers, W.R., Sharma, S.K., Wu, A.D., Nalin, C.M., Kaelin, W.G. Jr. (1996). Identification of a cyclin-cdk2 recognition motif present in substrates and p21-like cyclin-dependent kinase inhibitors. *Mol Cell Biol.*, 16: 6623–33

Araki, K., Nakajima, Y., Eto, K. & Ikeda, M.A. (2003). Distinct recruitment of E2F family members to specific E2F-binding sites mediates activation and repression of the E2F1 promoter. *Oncogene*, 22: 7632–7641

Bagella, L., Sun, A., Tonini, T., Abbadessa, G., Cottone, G., Paggi, M.G., De Luca, A., Claudio, P.P., Giordano, A. (2007). A small molecule based on the pRb2/p130 spacer domain leads to inhibition of cdk2 activity and cell cycle arrest. *Oncogene*, 26: 1829-39

Baldi, A., De Luca, A., Claudio, P.P., Baldi, F., Giordano, G.G., Tommasino, M., Paggi, M.G. & Giordano, A. (1995). The Rb2/p130 gene product is a nuclear protein whose phosphorylation is cycle regulated. *J Cell Biochem.*, 59: 402–408

Baldi, A., Esposito, V., De Luca, A., Howard, C.M., Mazzarella, G., Baldi, F., Caputi, M. & Giordano, A. (1996). Differential expression of the retinoblastoma gene family members pRb/p105, p107, and pRb2/p130 in lung cancer. *Clin Cancer Res.*, 2: 1239–45

Baylin, S.B. (2005). DNA methylation and gene silencing in cancer. *Nat Clin Pract Oncol.*, 2: S4–11

Baylin, S.B. & Herman, J.G. (2000). DNA hypermethylation in tumorigenesis: epigenetics joins genetics. *Trends Genet.*, 16: 168–174

Bellan, C., De Falco, G., Tosi, G.M., Lazzi, S., Ferrari, F., Morbini, G., Bartolomei, S., Toti, P., Mangiavacchi, P., Cevenini, G., Trimarchi, C., Cinti, C., Giordano, A., Leoncini, L., Tosi, P. & Cottier, H. (2002). Missing expression of pRb2/p130 in human retinoblastomas is associated with reduced apoptosis and lesser differentiation. *Invest Ophthalmol Vis Sci.*, 43: 3602–3608

Besson, A., Dowdy, S.F. & Roberts, J.M. (2008). CDK inhibitors: cell cycle regulators and beyond. *Dev Cell.*, 14: 159–69

Boehm, J.S. & Hahn, W.C. (2011). Towards systematic functional characterization of cancer genomes. *Nat Rev Genet.*, 12: 487–98

Bracken, A.P., Pasini, D., Capra, M., Prosperini, E., Colli, E. & Helin, K. (2003). EZH2 is downstream of the pRB-E2F pathway, essential for proliferation and amplified in cancer. *EMBO J.*, 22: 5323–35

Brehm A., Miska E.A., McCance D.J., Reid J.L., Bannister A.J. & Kouzarides T. (1998). Retinoblastoma protein recruits histone deacetylase to repress transcription. *Nature*, 391: 597–601

Burkhart, D.L. & Sage, J. (2008). Cellular mechanisms of tumour suppression by the retinoblastoma gene. *Nat Rev Cancer.*, 8: 671–82

Caldeira, S., De Villiers, E.M., Tommasino, M. (2000). Human papillomavirus E7 proteins stimulate proliferation independently of their ability to associate with retinoblastoma protein. *Oncogene*, 19: 821–826

Cánepa, E.T., Scassa, M.E., Ceruti, J.M., Marazita, M.C., Carcagno, A.L, Sirkin, P.F. & Ogara, MF. (2007). INK4 proteins, a family of mammalian CDK inhibitors with novel biological functions. *IUBMB Life*, 59: 419–26

Canhoto, A.J., Chestukhin, A., Litovchick, L., DeCaprio, J.A. (2000). Phosphorylation of the retinoblastoma-related protein p130 in growth-arrested cells. *Oncogene*, 19: 5116–5122

Caputi, M., Groeger, A.M., Esposito, V., De Luca, A., Masciullo, V., Mancini, A., Baldi, F., Wolner, E. & Giordano, A. (2002). Loss of pRb2/p130 expression is associated with unfavorable clinical outcome in lung cancer. *Clin Cancer Res.*, 8: 3850–6

Caracciolo, V., Reiss, K., Khalili, K., De Falco, G. & Giordano, A. (2006). Role of the interaction between large T antigen and Rb family members in the oncogenicity of JC virus. *Oncogene*, 25: 5294–301

Chen, H., Tsai, S. & Leone, G. (2009). Emerging roles of E2Fs in cancer: an exit from cell cycle control. *Nature Reviews Cancer*, 9: 785–797

Chestukhin, A., Litovchick, L., Rudich, K. & DeCaprio, JA. (2002). Nucleocytoplasmic shuttling of p130/RBL2: novel regulatory mechanism. *Mol Cell Biol.* 22: 453–68

Ciccolini, F., Di Pasquale, G., Carlotti, F., Crawford, L. & Tommasino, M. (1994). Functional studies of E7 proteins from different HPV types. *Oncogene*, 9: 2633–2638

Cinti, C., Leoncini, L., Nyongo, A., Ferrari, F., Lazzi, S., Bellan, C., Vatti, R., Zamparelli, A., Cevenini, G., Tosi, G.M., Claudio, P.P., Maraldi, N.M., Tosi, P. & Giordano, A. (2000). Genetic alterations of the retinoblastoma-related gene RB2/p130 identify different pathogenetic mechanisms in and among Burkitt's lymphoma subtypes. *Am J Pathol.*, 156: 751-60

Cinti, C., Macaluso, M. & Giordano, A. (2005). Tumor-specific exon 1 mutations could be the "hit event" predisposing Rb2/p130 gene to epigenetic silencing in lung cancer. *Oncogene*, 24:5821-6

Cirillo, D., Pentimalli, F. & Giordano, A. (2011). Peptides or Small Molecules? Different Approaches to Develop More Effective CDK Inhibitors. *Curr Med Chem.*,18: 2854-66

Clarke, A.R., Maandag, E.R., van Roon, M., van der Lugt, N.M., van der Valk, M., Hooper, M.L., Berns, A. & te Riele, H. (1992). Requirement for a functional Rb-1 gene in murine development. *Nature*, 359: 328-30

Classon, M., Salama, S., Gorka, C., Mulloy, R., Braun, P. & Harlow, E. (2000). Combinatorial roles for pRB, p107, and p130 in E2F-mediated cell cycle control. *Proc Natl Acad Sci USA*, 97: 10820-10825

Classon, M. & Dyson, N. (2001). p107 and p130: versatile proteins with interesting pockets. *Exp Cell Res.*, 264: 135-47

Claudio, P.P., Howard, C.M., Baldi, A., De Luca, A., Fu, Y., Condorelli, G., Sun, Y., Colburn, N., Calabretta, B. & Giordano, A. (1994). p130/pRb2 has growth suppressive properties similar to yet distinctive from those of retinoblastoma family members pRb and p107. *Cancer Res.*, 54: 5556-5560

Claudio, P.P., De Luca, A., Howard, C.M., Baldi, A., Firpo, E.J., Koff, A., Paggi, M.G. & Giordano, A. (1996). Functional analysis of pRb2/p130 interaction with cyclins. *Cancer Res.*, 56: 2003-2008

Claudio, P.P., Howard, C.M., Fu, Y., Cinti, C., Califano, L., Micheli, P., Mercer, E.W., Caputi, M. & Giordano, A. (2000a). Mutations in the retinoblastoma-related gene RB2/p130 in primary nasopharyngeal carcinoma. *Cancer Res.*, 60: 8-12

Claudio P.P., Howard C.M., Pacilio C., Cinti C., Romano G., Minimo C., Maraldi N.M., Minna J.D., Gelbert L., Leoncini L, Tosi G.M., Hicheli P., Caputi M., Giordano G.G. & Giordano A. (2000b). Mutations in the retinoblastoma-related gene RB2/p130 in lung tumors and suppression of tumor growth in vivo by retrovirus-mediated gene transfer. *Cancer Res.*, 60: 372-82

Coats, S., Whyte, P., Fero, M.L., Lacy, S., Chung, G., Randel, E., Firpo, E. & Roberts J.M. (1999). A new pathway for mitogen-dependent Cdk2 regulation uncovered in p27Kip1-deficient cells. *Curr. Biol.*, 9: 163-173

Cobrinik, D., Lee, M.H., Hannon, G., Mulligan, G., Bronson, R.T., Dyson, N., Harlow, E., Beach, D., Weinberg, R.A. & Jacks, T. (1996). Shared role of the pRB-related p130 and p107 proteins in limb development. *Genes Dev.*, 10: 1633-44

Cobrinik, D. (2005). Pocket proteins and cell cycle control. *Oncogene,* 24: 2796-809

Croce, C.M. (2008). Oncogenes and cancer. *The New England journal of medicine,* 358(5): 502-11

Dahiya, A., Gavin, M.R., Luo, R.X. & Dean, D.C. (2000). Role of the LXCXE binding site in Rb function. *Mol Cell Biol.*, 20: 6799-805

Dahiya, A., Wong, S., Gonzalo, S., Gavin, M. & Dean, D.C. (2001). Linking the Rb and Polycomb Pathways. *Mol Cell*, 8: 557-569

Dai, Y. & Grant S. (2004). Small molecule inhibitors targeting cyclin-dependent kinases as anticancer agents. *Curr Oncol Rep.*, 6: 123-30

D'Andrilli, G., Masciullo, V., Bagella, L., Tonini, T., Minimo, C., Zannoni, C.F. Giuntoli, R.L. 2nd, Carlson, J.A. Jr., Soprano, D.R., Soprano, K.J., Scambia, G. & Giordano, A. (2004). Frequent Loss of pRb2/p130 in Human Ovarian Carcinoma. *Clin Cancer Res.*, 10: 3098–3103

Dannenberg, J.H., van Rossum, A., Schuijff, L. & te Riele, H. (2000). Ablation of the Retinoblastoma gene family deregulates G1 control causing immortalization and increased cell turnover under growth-restricting conditions. *Genes Dev.*, 14: 3051–3064

de Cárcer, G., Pérez de Castro, I. & Malumbres, M. (2007). Targeting cell cycle kinases for cancer therapy. *Curr Med Chem.*, 14: 969–85

De Falco, G., Leucci, E., Lenze, D., Piccaluga, P.P., Claudio, P.P., Onnis, A., Cerino, G., Nyagol, J., Mwanda, W., Bellan, C., Hummel, M., Pileri, S., Tosi, P., Stein, H., Giordano, A. & Leoncini, L. (2007). Gene-expression analysis identifies novel RBL2/p130 target genes in endemic Burkitt lymphoma cell lines and primary tumors. *Blood*, 110: 1301–7

De Luca, A., MacLachlan, T.K., Bagella, L., Dean, C., Howard, C.M., Claudio, P.P., Baldi, A., Khalili, K. & Giordano, A. (1997). A unique domain of pRb2/p130 acts as an inhibitor of Cdk2 kinase activity. *J Biol Chem.*, 272: 20971–4

Dimova D.K. & Dyson N.J. (2005). The E2F transcriptional network: old acquaintances with new faces. *Oncogene*, 24: 2810–26

Dong, F., Cress, Jr. W.D., Agrawal, D. & Pledger, W.J. (1998). The Role of Cyclin D3-dependent Kinase in the Phosphorylation of p130 in Mouse BALB/c 3T3 Fibroblasts. *J Biol Chem.*, 273: 6190–6195

Du, W. & Pogoriler, J. (2006). Retinoblastoma family genes. *Oncogene*, 25: 5190–200

Dunaief, J.L., Strober, B.E., Guha, S., Khavari, P.A., Alin, K., Luban, J., Begemann, M., Crabtree, G.R. & Goff, S.P. (1994). The retinoblastoma protein and BRG1 form a complex and cooperate to induce cell cycle arrest. *Cell*, 79:119-130

Dunaief, J.L., King, A., Esumi, N., Eagen, M., Dentchev, T., Sung, C.H., Chen, S., & Zack, D.J. (2002). Protein Phosphatase 1 binds strongly to the retinoblastoma protein but not to p107 or p130 in vitro and in vivo. *Curr Eye Res.*, 24: 392–396

Ewen, M.E., Xing, Y.G., Lawrence, J.B. & Livingston, D.M. (1991). Molecular cloning, chromosomal mapping, and expression of the cDNA for p107, a retinoblastoma gene product-related protein. *Cell*, 66: 1155–64

Fan, S., Yuan, R., Ma, Y.X., Xiong, J., Meng, Q., Erdos, M., Zhao, J.N., Goldberg, I.D., Pestell, R.G. & Rosen, E.M. (2001). Disruption of BRCA1 LXCXE motif alters BRCA1 functional activity and regulation of RB family but not RB protein binding. *Oncogene*, 20: 4827–4841

Fearon, E. R. (1997.) Human cancer syndromes: Clues to the origin and nature of cancer. *Science*, 278: 1043–1050

Felsani, A., Mileo, A.M. & Paggi, M.G. (2006). Retinoblastoma family proteins as key targets of the small DNA virus oncoproteins. *Oncogene*, 25: 5277–85

Ferreira, R., Magnaghi-Jaulin, L., Robin, P., Harel-Bellan, A. & Trouche, D. (1998). The three members of the pocket proteins family share the ability to repress E2F activity through recruitment of a histone deacetylase. *Proc Natl Acad Sci USA*, 95: 10493–8

Ferreira, R., Naguibneva, I., Mathieu, M., Ait-Si-Ali, S., Robin, P., Pritchard, L.L. & Harel-Bellan, A. (2001). Cell cycle-dependent recruitment of HDAC-1 correlates with deacetylation of histone H4 on an Rb–E2F target promote. *EMBO Rep.*, 2: 794–799

Fiorentino, F.P., Macaluso, M., Miranda, F., Montanari, M., Russo, A., Bagella, L. & Giordano, A. (2011). CTCF and BORIS Regulate Rb2/p130 Gene Transcription: A Novel Mechanism and a New Paradigm for Understanding the Biology of Lung Cancer. *Mol Cancer Res.*, 9: 225–33

Fischer, P.M. (2004). The use of CDK inhibitors in oncology: a pharmaceutical perspective. *Cell Cycle*, 3: 742–6

Friend, S.H., Bernards, R., Rogelj, S., Weinberg, R.A,. Rapaport, J.M, Albert, D.M. & Dryja, T.P. (1986). A human DNA segment with properties of the gene that predisposes to retinoblastoma and osteosarcoma. *Nature*, 323: 643–646

Fung, Y.K., Murphree, A.L., T'Ang A,. Qian, J., Hinrichs, S.H. &. Benedict, W.F. (1987). Structural evidence for the authenticity of the human retinoblastoma gene. *Science*, 236: 1657-1661

Gaubatz, S.F., Lindeman, G.J., Ishida, S., Jakoi, L., Nevins, J.R., Livingston, D.M. & Rempel R.E. (2000). E2F4 and E2F5 Play an Essential Role in Pocket Protein–Mediated G1 Control. *Molecular Cell.*, 6: 729–735

Giordano, A., Rossi, A., Romano, G., Bagella, L. (2007a). Tumor suppressor pRb2/p130 gene and its derived product Spa310 spacer domain as perspective candidates for cancer therapy. *J Cell Physiol.*, 213: 403-6

Giordano, A., Bellacchio, E., Bagella, L. & Paggi M.G. (2007b). Interaction between the Cdk2/cyclin A complex and a small molecule derived from the pRb2/p130 spacer domain: a theoretical model. *Cell Cycle*, 6: 2591–3

Graña, X. & Reddy, E.P. (1995). Cell cycle control in mammalian cells: role of cyclins, cyclin dependent kinases (CDKs), growth suppressor genes and cyclin-dependent kinase inhibitors (CKIs). Oncogene, 1995 11(2): 211–9

Graña, X., Garriga, J. & Mayol, X. (1998). Role of the retinoblastoma protein family, pRB, p107 and p130 in the negative control of cell growth. *Oncogene*, 17: 3365–83

Hanahan, D. & Weinberg, R. A. (2000). The hallmarks of cancer. *Cell*, 100: 57-70

Hansen, K., Farkas, T., Lukas, J., Holm, K., Rönnstrand, L. & Bartek, J. (2001). Phosphorylation-dependent and -independent functions of p130 cooperate to evoke a sustained G1 block. *EMBO J.*, 20: 422–32

Harbour, J.W., Luo, R.X., Dei Santi, A., Postigo, A.A. & Dean, D.C. (1999). Cdk Phosphorylation Triggers Sequential Intramolecular Interactions that Progressively Block Rb Functions as Cells Move through G1. *Cell*, 98: 859–869

Heeg, S., Doebele M., von Werder, A. & Opitz, O.G. (2006). In vitro transformation models: modeling human cancer. *Cell Cycle*, 6: 630-4

Helin, K., Holm, K., Niebuhr, A., Eiberg, H., Tommerup, N., Hougaard, S., Poulsen, H.S., Spang-Thomsen, M. & Norgaard, P. (1997). Loss of the retinoblastoma protein-related p130 protein in small cell lung carcinoma. *Proc Natl Acad Sci USA*, 94: 6933–8

Helt, A.M. & Galloway, D.A. (2003). Mechanisms by which DNA tumor virus oncoproteins target the Rb family of pocket proteins. *Carcinogenesis*, 24: 159–169

Herceg, Z. & Hainaut, P. (2007). Genetic and epigenetic alterations as biomarkers for cancer detection, diagnosis and prognosis. *Molecular Oncology*, 1: 26–41

Herrmann, C.H., Su, L.K. & Harlow, E. (1991). Adenovirus E1A is associated with a serine/threonine protein kinase. *J Virol.*, 65: 5848–5859

Hong, F.D., Huang, H.J., To H., Young, L.J., Oro, A., Bookstein, R., Lee, E.Y. & Lee, W.H. (1989). Structure of the human retinoblastoma gene. *Proc Natl Acad Sci USA*, 86: 5502–5506

Hu, Q.J., Dyson, N. & Harlow, E. (1990). The regions of the retinoblastoma protein needed for binding to adenovirus E1A or SV40 large T antigen are common sites for mutations. *EMBO J.*, 9: 1147–1155

Hurford, R.K., Cobrinik, D., Lee, M.H. & Dyson, N. (1997). pRB and p107/p130 are required for the regulated expression of different sets of E2F responsive genes. *Genes Dev*, 11: 1447–1463

Iavarone, A. & Massague, J. (1999). E2F and histone deacetylase mediate transforming growth factor beta repression of cdc25A during keratinocyte cell cycle arrest. *Mol Cell Biol.*, 19: 916–922

Ichimura, K., Hanafusa, H., Takimoto, H., Ohgama, Y., Akagi, T. & Shimizu, K. (2000). Structure of the human retinoblastoma-related p107 gene and its intragenic deletion in a B-cell lymphoma cell line. *Gene*, 251: 37–43

Jones, D.L., Thompson, D.A. & Munger, K. (1997). Destabilization of the RB Tumor Suppressor Protein and Stabilization of p53 Contribute to HPV Type 16 E7-Induced Apoptosis. *Virology*, 239: 97–107

Jones, P. A. & Baylin, S.B. (2002). The fundamental role of epigenetic events in cancer. *Nat Rev Genet.*, 3: 415–28

Johnson, D.G., Schwarz, J.K., Cress, W.D. & Nevins, J.R. (1993). Expression of transcription factor E2F1 induces quiescent cells to enter S phase. *Nature*, 365: 349–352

Kadam, S. & Emerson, B.M. (2003). Transcriptional Specificity of Human SWI/SNF BRG1 and BRM Chromatin Remodeling Complexes. *Mol Cell.*, 11: 377–389

Kiess, M., Gill, R.M. & Hamel, P.A. (1995). Expression and activity of the retinoblastoma protein (pRB)-family proteins, p107 and p130, during L6 myoblast differentiation. *Cell Growth Differ.*, 6: 1287–1298

Knudson, A. (1971). Mutation and cancer: statistical study of retinoblastoma. *Proc Natl Acad Sci USA*, 68: 820–823

Knudson, A.G. (1985). Hereditary cancer, oncogenes, and antioncogenes. *Cancer Res.*, 45(4):1437–43

Knudson, A. G. (1997). Hereditary predisposition to cancer. *Ann. N. Y. Acad. Sci.*, 833: 58–67

Knudson, A. G. (2001). Two genetic hits (more or less) to cancer. *Nat. Rev. Cancer*, 1: 157-162

Kotake, Y., Cao ,R., Viatour, P., Sage, J., Zhang, Y. & Xiong, Y. (2007). pRB family proteins are required for H3K27 trimethylation and Polycomb repression complexes binding to and silencing p16INK4alpha tumor suppressor gene. *Genes Dev.*, 21: 49–54

Lacy, S. & Whyte, P. (1997). Identification of a p130 domain mediating interactions with cyclin A/cdk 2 and cyclin E/cdk 2 complexes. *Oncogene*, 14: 2395–2406

Lammens, T., Li, J., Leone, G. & De Veylder, L. (2009). Atypical E2Fs: new players in the E2F transcription factor family. *Trends Cell Biol.*, 19: 111–8

Lazzi, S., Bellan, C., De Falco, G., Cinti, C., Ferrari, F., Nyongo, A., Claudio, P.P., Tosi, G.M., Vatti, R., Gloghini, A., Carbone, A., Giordano, A., Leoncini, L. & Tosi, P. (2002). Expression of RB2/p130 tumor-suppressor gene in AIDS-related non-Hodgkin's lymphomas: Implications for disease pathogenesis. *Hum Pathol.*, 33: 723–731

Le Cam, L., Polanowska, J., Fabbrizio, E., Olivier, M., Philips, A., Ng Eaton, E., Classon, M., Geng, Y. & Sardet, C. (1999). Timing of cyclin E gene expression depends on the regulated association of a bipartite repressor element with a novel E2F complex. *EMBO J.*, 18: 1878–1890

Lee, W.H., Bookstein, R., Hong, F., Young, L.J., Shew, J.Y. & Lee, E.Y. (1987a). Human retinoblastoma susceptibility gene: cloning, identification, and sequence. *Science,* 235: 1394–1399

Lee, W.H., Shew, J.Y., Hong, F.D., Sery T.W., Donoso, L.A., Young, L.J., Bookstein, R. & Lee, E.Y (1987b). The retinoblastoma susceptibility gene encodes a nuclear phosphoprotein associated with DNA binding activity. *Nature,* 329: 642–645

Lee, J.O., Russo, A.A. & Pavletich, N.P. (1998). Structure of the retinoblastoma tumour-suppressor pocket domain bound to a peptide from HPV E7. *Nature,* 39: 859–65

Lee, C., Chang, J.H., Lee, H.S. & Cho, Y. (2002). Structural basis for the recognition of the E2F transactivation domain by the retinoblastoma tumor suppressor. *Genes Dev,* 16: 3199–3212

Lees, E. (1995). Cyclin dependent kinase regulation. *Curr Opin Cell Biol.,* 7: 773–80

Levine, A.J. & Puzio-Kuter, A.M. (2010). The control of the metabolic switch in cancers by oncogenes and tumor suppressor genes. *Science,* 330:1340–4

Li, Y., Graham, C., Lacy, S., Duncan, A.M. & Whyte, P. (1993). The adenovirus E1A-associated 130-kD protein is encoded by a member of the retinoblastoma gene family and physically interacts with cyclins A and E. *Genes Dev.,* 7: 2366–77

Liu, H., Dibling, B., Spike, B., Dirlam, A. & Macleod, K. (2004). New roles for the RB tumor suppressor protein. *Curr. Opin. Genet. Dev.,* 14: 55–64

Liu, D.X., Nath, N., Chellappan, S.P. & Greene, L.A. (2005). Regulation of neuron survival and death by p130 and associated chromatin modifiers. *Genes Dev.,* 19: 719–732

Ludlow, J.W., Glendening, C.L., Livingston, D.M. & DeCarprio, J.A. (1993). Specific enzymatic dephosphorylation of the retinoblastoma protein. *Mol Cell Biol.,* 13: 367–372

Macaluso, M., Cinti, C., Russo, G., Russo, A. & Giordano, A. (2003). pRb2/p130-E2F4/5-HDAC1-SUV39H1-p300 and pRb2/p130-E2F4/5-HDAC1-SUV39H1-DNMT1 multimolecular complexes mediate the transcription of estrogen receptor-in breast cancer. *Oncogene,* 22: 3511–3517

Macaluso, M., Montanari, M. & Giordano, A. (2006). Rb family proteins as modulators of gene expression and new aspects regarding the interaction with chromatin remodeling enzymes. *Oncogene,* 25: 5263–7

Magnaghi-Jaulin, L., Groisman, R., Naguibneva, I., Robin, P., Lorain, S., Le Villain, J.P., Troalen, F., Trouche, D. & Harel-Bellan, A. (1998). Retinoblastoma protein represses transcription by recruiting a histone deacetylase. *Nature,* 391:601–5

Malumbres, M. & Barbacid, M. (2009). Cell cycle, CDKs and cancer: a changing paradigm. *Nat Rev Cancer,* 2009 9: 153–66

Mayol, X. & Grana, X. (1998). The p130 pocket protein: keeping order at cell cycle exit/re-entrance transitions. *Front Biosci.,* 3: d11–24

Mayol, X., Grana, X., Baldi, A., Sang, N., Hu, Q. & Giordano, A. (1993). Cloning of a new member of the retinoblastoma gene family (pRb2) which binds to the E1A transforming domain. *Oncogene,* 8: 2561–2566

Mayol, X., Garriga, J. & Grana, X. (1995). Cell cycle-dependent phosphorylation of the retinoblastoma-related protein p130. *Oncogene,* 11: 801–808

Mayol, X. & Graña, X. (1997). pRB, p107 and p130 as transcriptional regulators: role in cell growth and differentiation. *Prog Cell Cycle Res.*, 3: 157–69

McDonald, E.R. 3rd & El-Deiry, W.S. (2000). Cell cycle control as a basis for cancer drug development. *Int J Oncol.*, 16: 871–86

Milde-Langosch, K., Goemann, C., Methner, C., Rieck, G., Bamberger, A.M. & Loning, T. (2001). Expression of Rb2/p130 in breast and endometrial cancer: correlations with hormone receptor status. *Br J Cancer*, 85: 546–551

Moberg, K., Starz, M.A. & Lees, J.A. (1996). E2F-4 switches from p130 to p107 and pRB in response to cell cycle reentry. *Mol Cell Biol.*, 16: 1436–1449

Morgan, D.O. (1995). Principles of CDK regulation. *Nature*, 374: 131–4

Morgan, D.O. (1997). Cyclin-dependent kinases: engines, clocks, and microprocessors. *Annu. Rev. Cell. Dev. Biol.*, 13: 261-291

Morrison, A.J., Sardet, C. & Herrera, R.E. (2002). Retinoblastoma protein transcriptional repression through histone deacetylation of a single nucleosome. *Mol. Cell. Biol.*, 22: 856–865

Mulligan, G.J., Wong, J. & Jacks, T. (1998). p130 is dispensable in peripheral T lymphocytes: evidence for functional compensation by p107 and pRB. *Mol Cell Biol.*, 18: 206–20

Münger, K., Basile, J.R., Duensing, S., Eichten, A., Gonzalez, S.L., Grace, M. & Zacny, V.L. (2001). Biological activities and molecular targets of the human papillomavirus E7 oncoprotein. *Oncogene*, 20: 7888–7898

Murphree, A.L. & Benedict, W.F. (1984). Retinoblastoma: clues to human oncogenesis. *Science*, 223: 1028–33

Mutti, L., De Luca, A., Claudio, P.P., Convertino, G., Carbone, M. & Giordano, A. (1998). Simian virus 40-like DNA sequences and large-T antigen-retinoblastoma family protein pRb2/p130 interaction in human mesothelioma. *Dev Biol Stand.*, 94: 47–53

Napolitano, G., Majello, B. & Lania. L. (2002). Role of cyclinT/Cdk9 complex in basal and regulated transcription. *Int J Oncol.*, 21: 171–7

Nevins, J.R. (1998). Toward an understanding of the functional complexity of the E2F and retinoblastoma families. *Cell Growth Differ.*, 9: 585–93

Nielsch, U., Fognani, C. & Babiss, L.E. (1991). Adenovirus E1A-p105(Rb) protein interactions play a direct role in the initiation but not the maintenance of the rodent cell transformed phenotype. *Oncogene*, 6: 1031–1036

Paggi, M.G., Baldi, A., Bonetto, F. & Giordano, A. (1996). Retinoblastoma protein family in cell cycle and cancer: a review. *J Cell Biochem.*, 62(3):418–30

Polanowska, J., Fabbrizio, E., Le Cam, L., Trouche, D., Emiliani, S., Herrera, R. & Sardet C. (2001). The periodic down regulation of Cyclin E gene expression from exit of mitosis to end of G1 is controlled by a deacetylase- and E2F-associated bipartite repressor element. *Oncogene*, 20: 4115–4127

Putzer, B.M., Rumpf, H., Rega, S., Brockmann, D. & Esche, H. (1997). E1A 12S and 13S of the transformation-defective adenovirus type 12 strain CS-1 inactivate proteins of the RB family, permitting transactivation of the E2F-dependent promoter. *J Virol.*, 71: 9538–9548

Rayman, J.B., Takahashi, Y., Indjeian, V.B., Dannenberg, J.H., Catchpole, S., Watson, R.J., te Riele, H. & Dynlacht, B.D. (2002). E2F mediates cell cycle-dependent transcriptional repression in vivo by recruitment of an HDAC1/mSin3B corepressor complex. *Genes Dev.*, 16: 933–947

Ross, J.F., Liu X. & Dynlacht, B.D. (1999). Mechanism of transcriptional repression of E2F by the retinoblastoma tumor suppressor protein. *Mol Cell.*, 3:195-205

Ruiz, S., Segrelles, C., Bravo, A., Santos, M., Perez, P., Leis, H., Jorcano, J.L. & Paramio, J.M. (2003). Abnormal epidermal differentiation and impaired epithelial-mesenchymal tissue interactions in mice lacking the retinoblastoma relatives p107 and p130. *Development*, 130: 2341–2353

Rumpf, H., Esche, H. & Kirch, H.C. (1999). Two Domains within the Adenovirus Type 12 E1A UniqueSpacer Have Disparate Effects on the Interaction of E1A with P105-Rb and the Transformation of Primary Mouse Cells. *Virology*, 257: 45–53

Sage, J., Mulligan, G.J., Attardi, L.D., Miller, A., Chen, S., Williams, B., Theodorou, E. & Jacks, T. (2000). Targeted disruption of the three Rb-related genes leads to loss of G1 control and immortalization. *Genes Dev.*, 14: 3037–3050

Schaffer, B.E., Park, K.S., Yiu, G., Conklin, J.F., Lin, C., Burkhart, D.L., Karnezis, A.N., Sweet-Cordero, E.A. & Sage, J. (2010). Loss of p130 accelerates tumor development in a mouse model for human small-cell lung carcinoma. *Cancer Res.*, 70: 3877–83

Shapiro, G.I. (2006). Cyclin-dependent kinase pathways as targets for cancer treatment. *J Clin Oncol.*, 24: 1770–83

Sidle, A., Palaty, C., Dirks, P., Wiggan, O., Kiess, M., Gill, R.M., Wong, A.K. & Hamel, P.A. (1996). Activity of the retinoblastoma family proteins, pRB, p107, and p130, during cellular proliferation and differentiation. *Crit Rev Biochem Mol Biol.*, 31: 237–271

Simpson, D.S., Mason-Richie, N.A., Gettler, C.A. & Wikenheiser-Brokamp, K.A. (2009). Retinoblastoma family proteins have distinct functions in pulmonary epithelial cells in vivo critical for suppressing cell growth and tumorigenesis. *Cancer Res.*, 69: 8733-41

Smith, E.J., Leone, G., DeGregori, J., Jakoi, L. & Nevins, J.R. (1996). The accumulation of an E2F-p130 transcriptional repressor distinguishes a G0 cell state from a G1 cell state. *Mol Cell Biol.*, 16: 6965–6976

Smith, E.J., Leone, G. & Nevins, J.R. (1998). Distinct mechanisms control the accumulation of the Rb-related p107 and p130 proteins during cell growth. *Cell Growth Differ.*, 9: 297–303

Stiegler, P., De Luca, A., Bagella, L. & Giordano, A. (1998). The COOH-terminal region of pRb2/p130 binds to histone deacetylase 1 (HDAC1), enhancing transcriptional repression of the E2F-dependent cyclin A promoter. *Cancer Res.*, 58: 5049-52

Stiegler, P. & Giordano, A. (1999). Role of pRB2/p130 in cellular growth regulation. *Anal Quant Cytol Histol.*, 21: 363–366

Stiegler, P. & Giordano, A. (2001). The family of retinoblastoma proteins. *Crit Rev Eukaryot Gene Expr.*, 11: 59–76

Sun, A., Bagella, L., Tutton, S., Romano, G. & Giordano, A. (2007). From G0 to S phase: A view of the roles played by the retinoblastoma (Rb) family members in the Rb-E2F pathway. *J Cell Biochem.*, 102: 1400–4

Takahashi, Y., Rayman, J.B. & Dynlacht, B.D. (2000). Analysis of promoter binding by the E2F and pRB families in vivo: distinct E2F proteins mediate activation and repression. *Genes Dev.*, 14: 804–816

Taubert, S., Gorrini, C., Frank, S.R., Parisi, T., Fuchs, M., Chan, H.M., Livingston, D.M. & Amati, B. (2004). E2F-Dependent Histone Acetylation and Recruitment of the Tip60 Acetyltransferase Complex to Chromatin in Late G1. *Mol. Cell. Biol.*, 24: 4546–4556

Tedesco, D., Lukas, J. & Reed, S.I. (2002). The pRb-related protein p130 is regulated by phosphorylation-dependent proteolysis via the protein-ubiquitin ligase SCF(Skp2). *Genes Dev.*, 16: 2946–57

Tonini T., Bagella L., D'Andrilli G., Claudio P.P. & Giordano A. (2004). Ezh2 reduces the ability of HDAC1-dependent pRb2/p130 transcriptional repression of cyclin A. *Oncogene*, 23: 4930–7

Tonini, T., D'Andrilli, G., Fucito, A., Gaspa, L. & Bagella, L. (2008). Importance of Ezh2 polycomb protein in tumorigenesis process interfering with the pathway of growth suppressive key elements. *J Cell Physiol.*, 214: 295–300

Vanderluit, J.L., Ferguson, K.L., Nikoletopoulou, V., Parker, M., Ruzhynsky, V., Alexson, T., McNamara, S.M., Park, D.S., Rudnicki M. & Slack R.S. (2004). p107 regulates neural precursor cells in the mammalian brain. *J. Cell Biol.*, 166: 853–863

Vuocolo, S., Purev, E., Zhang, D., Bartek, J., Hansen, K., Soprano, D.R. & Soprano, K.J. (2003). Protein Phosphatase 2A Associates with Rb2/p130 and Mediates Retinoic Acid-induced Growth Suppression of Ovarian Carcinoma Cells. *J. Biol. Chem.*, 278: 41881–41889

Wells, J., Boyd, K.E., Fry, C.J., Bartley, S.M. & Farnham, P.J. (2000). Target Gene Specificity of E2F and Pocket Protein Family Members in Living Cells *Mol. Cell. Biol.*, 20: 5797–5807

Whittaker, S.R., Walton, M.I., Garrett, M.D. & Workman, P. (2004). The Cyclin-dependent kinase inhibitor CYC202 (R-roscovitine) inhibits retinoblastoma protein phosphorylation, causes loss of Cyclin D1, and activates the mitogen-activated protein kinase pathway. *Cancer Res.*, 64: 262–72

Whyte, P., Williamson, N.M. & Harlow, E. (1989). Cellular targets for transformation by the adenovirus E1A proteins. *Cell*, 56: 67–75

Woo, M.S., Sánchez, I. & Dynlacht, B.D.(1997). p130 and p107 use a conserved domain to inhibit cellular cyclin-dependent kinase activity. *Mol Cell Biol.*, 17: 3566–79

Xiao, B., Spencer, J., Clements, A., Ali-Khan, N., Mittnacht, S., Broceno, C., Burghammer, M., Perrakis A., Marmorstein, R., & Gamblin, S.J. (2003). Crystal structure of the retinoblastoma tumor suppressor protein bound to E2F and the molecular basis of its regulation. *Proc Natl Acad Sci USA*, 100: 2363–2368

Yeung, R.S., Bell, D.W., Testa, J.R., Mayol, X., Baldi, A., Graña, X., Klinga-Levan, K., Knudson, A.G. & Giordano, A. (1993). The retinoblastoma-related gene, RB2, maps to human chromosome 16q12 and rat chromosome 19. *Oncogene*, 8: 3465–8

Zhang, H.S., Gavin, M., Dahiya, A., Postigo, A.A., Ma, D., Luo, R.X., Harbour, J.W., & Dean, D.C. (2000). Exit from G1 and S Phase of the Cell Cycle Is Regulated by Repressor Complexes Containing HDAC-Rb-hSWI/SNF and Rb-hSWI/SNF. *Cell*, 101: 79–8

Zheng, N., Fraenkel, E., Pabo, C.O., Pavletich, N.P. (1999). "Structural basis of DNA recognition by the heterodimeric cell cycle transcription factor E2F-DP". *Genes Dev.*, 13: 666–7

Zhu, L., van den Heuvel, S., Helin, K., Fattaey, A., Ewen, M., Livingston, D., Dyson, N. & Harlow, E. (1993). Inhibition of cell proliferation by p107, a relative of the retinoblastoma protein. *Genes Dev.*, 7: 1111–1125

Zhu L., Harlow E. & Dynlacht BD. (1995). p107 uses a p21CIP1-related domain to bind cyclin/cdk2 and regulate interactions with E2F. *Genes Dev.*, 9: 1740–1752

Zhu, W., Giangrande, P.H. & Nevins, J.R. (2004). E2Fs link the control of G1/S and G2/M transcription. *EMBO J.*, 23: 4615–4626

7

Significance of Retinoblastoma Protein in Survival and Differentiation of Cerebellar Neurons

Jaya Padmanabhan
Department of Molecular Medicine, Tampa, FL
USF Health Byrd Alzheimer's Institute, Tampa, FL
USA

1. Introduction

During development of the nervous system an excess number of neural progenitor cells are generated and approximately half of these cells are eliminated by programmed cell death (PCD) or apoptosis (Farinelli and Greene, 1996; Jacobson et al., 1997; Oppenheim, 1991; Raff, 1992; Raff et al., 1993). The apoptosis and elimination of the excess number of precursor cells enable the proper synaptic integration of the surviving cells and development of the central nervous system (CNS). Survival of the neurons in the CNS requires trophic support and electrical activity and upon withdrawal or depletion of these factors the neurons undergo apoptosis (Barde et al., 1987; Biffo et al., 1994; D'Mello et al., 1997; D'Mello et al., 1993; D'Mello et al., 2000; Galli et al., 1995; Levi-Montalcini, 1987; Miller and Johnson, 1996). Among the growth factors that support neuronal survival and differentiation are neurotrophic growth factor (NGF), brain derived neurotrophic factor (BDNF), neurotrophin 3 and 4 (NT3 and NT4), insulin and insulin like growth factors (IGF), glial derived neurotrophic factor (GDNF), basic fibroblast growth factor (bFGF), and ciliary neurotrophic factor (CNTF) (Ardelt et al., 1994; Barde, 1994; de Pablo et al., 1990a; de Pablo et al., 1990b; Ferrari et al., 1989; Ferrer et al., 1998; Hynes et al., 1994; Kalcheim et al., 1987; Knusel et al., 1990; Levi-Montalcini, 1987; Lindholm et al., 1993; Magal et al., 1993; Rabacchi et al., 1999; Rakowicz et al., 2002; Serrano et al., 1990; Tuttle et al., 1994; Zhang et al., 1997).

Many neurological diseases such as Alzheimer's, tauopathies, Parkinson's etc., show neuronal loss in specific areas of the brain (Burke, 1998; Cotman and Anderson, 1995; Cotman and Su, 1996; Forloni, 1993; Gorman et al., 1996; Hajimohamadreza and Treherne, 1997; Hartmann and Hirsch, 2001; Honig and Rosenberg, 2000; Jellinger, 2001; Johnson, 1994; Savitz and Rosenbaum, 1998; Yanagisawa, 2000; Yuan and Yankner, 2000). Although a number of signaling pathways have been implicated in the apoptosis observed in the brains it is difficult to determine whether inhibition of these pathways has any effect on neuronal survival *in vivo*. Therefore, in order to understand the *in vivo* mechanisms involved in neuronal apoptosis, researchers mainly use either transgenic mouse models or *in vitro* cultures of dissociated primary neurons or organotypic slice cultures from different brain regions from rodents. The mechanisms by which the different types of neurons undergo apoptosis vary, and it depends on the type of insult as well as the type of neurons involved. For example, studies in sympathetic ganglia have shown that growth factor withdrawal and oxidative stress-induced apoptosis is associated with caspase activation and cyclin D1 expression (Freeman et al., 1994; Stefanis et al., 1998; Troy et al., 1997; Troy et al., 1996). Inhibitors of caspases such as z-DEVD-FMK and z-VAD-FMK protected these neurons from undergoing apoptosis thereby confirming that indeed caspase activation is involved in cell death. Similarly insults such as Aβ treatment, growth factor deprivation and treatment with DNA damaging agents induce apoptosis in cortical neurons, which is associated with activation of caspases as well as cell cycle regulatory proteins (Park et al., 1997a; Park et al., 1997b; Park et al., 1998a; Park et al., 1998b; Stefanis et al., 1999; Troy et al., 2000; Troy et al., 2001). Activation of cell cycle regulatory mechanisms have also been implicated in cerebellar granule neurons (CGNs) undergoing activity withdrawal-induced apoptosis (Konishi and Bonni, 2003b; Konishi et al., 2002; O'Hare et al., 2000; Padmanabhan et al., 1999).

It is now established that in neurons subjected to apoptotic insults, retinoblastoma protein (Rb) undergoes cdk-mediated phosphorylation which leads to its inactivation and dissociation from E2F (Boutillier et al., 1999; O'Hare et al., 2000; Padmanabhan et al., 1999; Park et al., 1997a; Park et al., 1997b; Park et al., 1998a; Sakai et al., 1999). Dissociated E2Fs induce transactivation of specific proapoptotic genes and apoptosis in different types of cells including neurons. In addition to transcriptional activation, derepression of proapoptotic genes is also implicated in neurons undergoing apoptosis. For example, studies have shown that the transcription factors B-Myb and C-myb are induced in cortical neurons subjected to growth factor withdrawal and DNA damage mediated apoptosis (Liu et al., 2004; Liu and Greene, 2001). It was found that the antisense RNA-mediated down regulation of B-myb and C-myb protected neurons from undergoing apoptosis and overexpression of these transcription factors was sufficient to induce apoptosis. This suggests that cell cycle activation in neurons induce dissociation of Rb/E2F complex leading to derepression and transactivation of proapoptotic genes.

This chapter mainly focuses on the mechanisms involved in neuronal apoptosis in cerebellum. Within the developing brain, cerebellar cortex has been extensively used for studying neuronal survival and apoptosis. The cerebellum plays a major role in movement, motor coordination, learning and cognitive function (Wechsler-Reya and Scott, 2001). It contains different types of neurons, of which Purkinje neuron is the most elaborate with a large cell body and vast dendritic tree. Due to the abundance of cerebellar granule neurons (CGNs) they have been used widely to study molecular mechanisms of neurodegeneration. The granule neurons differentiate into mature neurons when cultured in the presence of appropriate growth factors or when supported by depolarizing concentrations of KCl (D'Mello et al., 1997; D'Mello et al., 1993; Miller and Johnson, 1996). Growth factors that usually support survival of CGN are serum and IGF-1. Treatment of CGNs with high concentrations of KCl (25 to 30 mM) induces electrical activity and membrane depolarization, which allows Ca2+ entry through voltage sensitive calcium channels (Catterall, 2000; Konishi and Bonni, 2003b). Growth factor removal and KCl withdrawal induce neuronal apoptosis in CGNs, which involves different types of signaling pathways. This chapter mainly focuses on the involvement of cell cycle regulatory proteins in cerebellar granule and Purkinje neuron apoptosis and highlights the importance of functional retinoblastoma protein in survival and maintenance of differentiated neurons.

2. Retinoblastoma protein

Retinoblastoma protein (Rb) is a negative regulator of cell cycle progression and is known as the master regulator of cell cycle, differentiation, senescence and apoptosis (Chen et al., 1995; Dasgupta et al., 2006; Herwig and Strauss, 1997; Knudsen et al., 2000; Lee et al., 1995; Riley et al., 1994; Wang, 1997; Wang et al., 1994; Weinberg, 1989a, b, 1990, 1991, 1995). It belongs to a family of proteins known as pocket proteins, which include p107 and p130. These proteins bind to the early transcription factors (E2Fs) and control the G1/S transition of cells. Rb associates with several members of the E2F family and inhibits transactivation of E2F-responsive genes. Among the E2F family members (E2Fs 1 through 8) E2Fs 1, 2, and 3 are transcriptional activators and have been shown to associate with Rb. The binding of Rb to E2F depends on the phosphorylation state of Rb (Angus et al., 2002; Chellappan et al., 1991; Hiebert et al., 1992; Nevins et al., 1991). A cell, upon receipt of growth factor or different proliferative signals, induce expression of cyclin D in the early G1 phase and cyclin E in the later G1 phase. These cyclins associate with the respective cyclin-dependent kinases (cdk). Cdk4 and cdk6 associate with cyclin D1 while cdk2 interacts with cyclin E. The cyclin-cdk complex induces phosphorylation of Rb leading to its inactivation and dissociation from E2F which results in G1/S checkpoint release and E2F-dependent transcriptional activation (Figure 1). Thus, functional retinoblastoma protein plays a major role in control of cell division and loss of its function by mutation, phosphorylation or degradation leads to uncontrolled cell division and tumorigenesis. After G1/S checkpoint release, further progression of cells through S and G2/M phases are brought about by cyclin A/cdk2 (S-phase) and cyclin B/cdc2 (cdk1) complexes, respectively. In addition to the cdks, the *in vivo* inhibitors of cdks (CKIs) such as p16, p21, p27 and p57 also play a role in cell cycle control (Besson et al., 2008). Thus, cell cycle is tightly regulated by the combined efforts of cyclins, cdks, cyclin-dependent kinase inhibitors (CKIs) and Rb.

In addition to its anti-proliferative role, retinoblastoma protein can also function as an anti-apoptotic factor. Rb exerts its growth-inhibitory effects mainly by binding and inhibiting transactivation of E2F family of transcription factors (Chellappan et al., 1991; Dasgupta et al., 2004; Nevins et al., 1991; Stevaux and Dyson, 2002). Among these transcription factors, E2F1 has been implicated in not only S-phase entry but also apoptosis induction through the p53 and p73 pathways (Irwin et al., 2000; Lissy et al., 2000; Zaika et al., 2001). Overexpression of Rb inhibits E2F1-mediated apoptosis. It has been suggested that the increased apoptosis observed in Rb null mice is brought about mainly by increased E2F1 activity. Studies by Chellappan and colleagues have shown that in addition to the cyclins and cdks, non-cyclin dependent kinases can also phosphorylate and inactivate Rb (Dasgupta et al., 2004; Nath et al., 2003; Wang et al., 1999a; Wang et al., 1999b). For example, during mitogenic signaling, Raf1 directly interacts with and phosphorylates Rb. Analysis of Rb-associated mechanisms in cells undergoing apoptosis showed an interaction of Rb with kinases such as p38 MAP kinase and apoptosis signal regulating kinase 1 (ASK1) (Dasgupta et al., 2004). This suggests that in addition to the cdks Rb can be phosphorylated and inactivated by non-cyclin-dependent kinases as well.

Several viral oncoproteins such as the SV-40 large T-antigen (T-Ag), E1A of the adenovirus and E7 of the human papilloma virus type 16 have been shown to bind Rb through an LXCXE motif. Interaction of Rb with viral oncoproteins lead to dissociation of Rb from E2F and induction of E2F-dependent gene expression (Chellappan et al., 1992; Chellappan et al.,

1991; Hiebert et al., 1992; Nevins et al., 1991). Loss of Rb function leads to an increase in p53 activity via an E2F-dependent induction of ARF family of proteins. ARF induces degradation of MDM2 and stabilization of p53 (Kamijo et al., 1998; Pomerantz et al., 1998; Tao and Levine, 1999; Weber et al., 2000; Zhang et al., 1998). This is one of the mechanisms by which Rb induces p53-dependent apoptosis in non-transformed cells. Similarly, human cytomegalovirus (HCMV) has been shown to inhibit the Rb-E2F association. The HCMV-mediated Rb inactivation was not inhibited by the cdk inhibitors roscovitine, olomoucine or flavopiridol. *In vitro* and *in vivo* studies have shown that HCMV-mediated Rb phosphorylation is brought about by UL97, an HCMV protein kinase, and inhibition or inactivation of this kinase can prevent Rb phosphorylation (Hume et al., 2008).

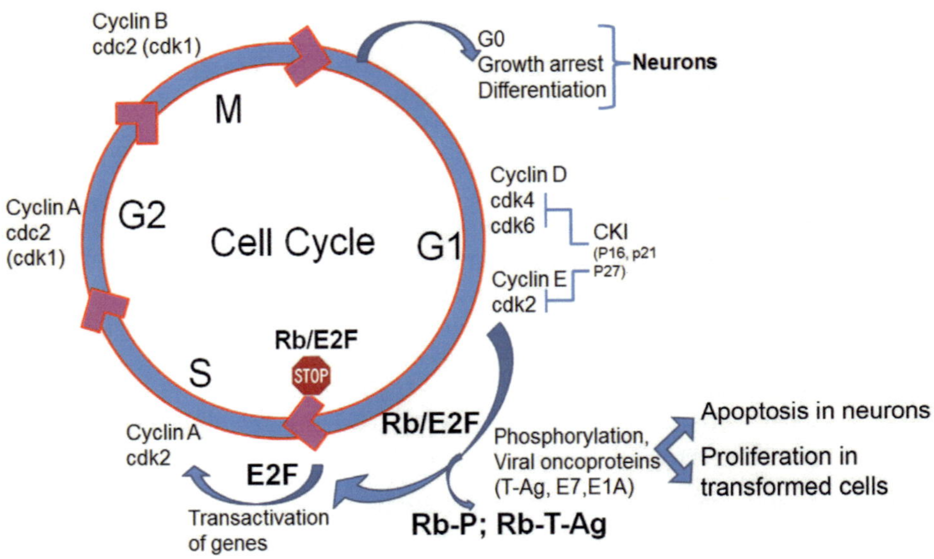

Fig. 1. Retinoblastoma (Rb) protein and cell cycle: In resting cells Rb associates with E2F and prevents (STOP) transition of cells through the G1→S checkpoint. Upon receipt of growth factors or proliferative signals, cyclins and cdks are activated leading to phosphorylation of Rb (Rb-P) and release of Rb from E2F. In the early G1 phase cyclin D associates with cdk4 or cdk6 and in the late G1 phase cyclin E associates with cdk2 to induce phosphorylation and inactivation of Rb. The activities of the cdks are regulated by cyclin-dependent kinase inhibitors (CKI). These CKIs, such as p16, p21 and p27, inhibit cdks from phosphorylating and inactivating Rb. In addition to phosphorylation, binding of viral oncoproteins such as SV-40 large T-antigen (T-Ag), E1A of adenovirus and E7 of papilloma virus can also inactivate Rb. Binding of these oncoproteins to Rb (example, Rb-T-Ag) releases Rb from E2F resulting in transactivation of E2F-dependent genes needed for cell proliferation. Once the cells pass through the G1/S checkpoint, further progression through cell cycle is made possible by cyclin A/cdk2 in S phase and Cylin B/cdc2 (cdk1) in the G2-M phase. Fully developed mature neurons are differentiated cells and are retained in the G0 phase of the cell cycle. Unlike proliferating cells which undergo transformation and uncontrolled proliferation upon Rb inactivation, neurons undergo neurodegeneration and apoptosis demonstrating the importance of Rb in maintenance of healthy differentiated neurons.

3. Retinoblastoma protein and neuronal survival

In addition to its function in control of cell cycle, Rb has been shown to be important in development and survival of neurons (Athanasiou et al., 1998; Feddersen et al., 1995; Feddersen et al., 1997; Hoglinger et al., 2007; Padmanabhan et al., 2007). Although it is known that precursor cells can divide and the newly formed daughter cells can migrate and differentiate into mature neurons, the ability of mature neurons to divide is debatable. Mature neurons are usually maintained in the G_0 or the resting phase of the cell cycle and respond to cell cycle activation by undergoing apoptosis rather than transformation. This is further supported by the fact that there are rarely any cases of tumors that originate from mature neurons. Several lines of evidence indicate that neuronal development and survival requires the presence of functional Rb in the nervous system. Mice lacking Rb show defects in neurogenesis and die embryonically at day 16 (Clarke et al., 1992; Jacks et al., 1992; Lee et al., 1992). This shows that Rb is important for proper exit of immature precursor cells from cell cycle and generation of mature differentiated neurons, and in the absence of Rb they attempt to reenter cell cycle but undergo neurodegeneration and apoptosis.

4. Degeneration of cerebellar neurons

4.1 Cerebellar granule neurons

Cerebellar granule neurons (CGN) when cultured in the presence of serum and depolarizing concentrations of KCl (25 mM) acquire characteristics of fully differentiated mature neurons similar to those present *in vivo* (Galli et al., 1995). Upon lowering the concentration of KCl to 5 mM these neurons undergo apoptosis. Apoptosis in CGN is prevented by treatment with IGF-1, cyclic AMP, forskolin and inhibitors of transcription and translation (D'Mello et al., 1997; D'Mello et al., 1993; Miller and Johnson, 1996; Padmanabhan et al., 1999). The protection of cells by transcriptional inhibitors point to the fact that under apoptotic conditions the transcriptional machinery is activated. Since cell cycle dependent mechanisms are under transcriptional regulation it was hypothesized that neuronal apoptosis may be associated with deregulation of cell cycle.

Although neuronal apoptosis has been shown to be associated with activation of caspases, no significant protection was observed by caspase inhibitors upon activity withdrawal-induced apoptosis in CGNs. This led to the analysis of the role of cell cycle regulatory proteins in this apoptosis paradigm (Padmanabhan et al., 2007). Neurons were deprived of KCl in the presence of inhibitors of cdks and their survival was examined at different time points. It was found that the cdk inhibitors could provide significant protection of rat CGN from KCl deprivation induced apoptosis even when the caspase acitivity was high (Padmanabhan et al., 1999). The discrepancy in the results from different laboratories could be explained by the age of the culture, origin of the cells (mouse vs rats), or the culture conditions. It is possible that lowering the KCl concentrations to 5 mM without withdrawal of serum may use a different mechanism to induce apoptosis compared to that induced by withdrawal of both serum and KCl. It is known that KCl withdrawal is associated with induction in caspase activity and treatment of the neurons with a general caspase inhibitor can significantly prevent the increase in activity. This suggests that irrespective of the status of caspases in the cells, transcriptional activation clearly leads to KCl withdrawal-induced cell death in CGN. Analysis of cyclin D1 and cyclin E showed that these cylcins are normally present in the CGNs. Upon KCl withdrawal, the cells begin to undergo a time-dependent apoptosis and the expression of these cyclins is induced. Immunostaining analysis revealed that neurons undergoing apoptosis accumulate cyclin D1 in their nucleus which is indicative of its role in activation of cell cycle (Padmanabhan et al., 1999). This result is different from what has been observed in sympathetic neurons wherein the expression of cyclin D1 is non-detectable under non-apoptotic conditions and is detectable only upon growth factor deprivation-induced apoptosis. This shows that the gene expression patterns vary between neurons from different regions and therefore may respond differently to diverse external cues.

Immunoprecipitation and kinase activity assays showed that apoptosis in CGN is associated with an induction in cyclin D1 and cyclin E-associated kinase activities (Padmanabhan et al., 1999). *In vivo* inhibitors of cdks such as p16, p21, p27 and p57 (CKIs) regulate the activities of cdks. It was found that the neurons undergoing apoptosis show a time-dependent decrease in p27 levels (Martin-Romero et al., 2000; Padmanabhan et al., 1999). Decreased p27 levels in turn, enhance the cdk activity further and enable cdks to phosphorylate and inactivate Rb resulting in dissociation of Rb from E2F. This leads to enhanced E2F-dependent transactivation or derepression of proapoptotic genes. Analysis of the neurons showed that Rb phosphorylation and degradation are enhanced in cells undergoing apoptosis (Padmanabhan et al., 1999). Since Rb is the major regulator of G1→S phase transition, this observation indicates that the neurons are forced to exit the G0 phase and re-enter the cell cycle. Although the neurons exit the resting phase of the cell cycle they do not undergo cell division or transformation but instead undergo apoptosis.

Treatment of the neurons with inhibitors of cdks protected CGNs from KCl withdrawal-induced apoptosis (Padmanabhan et al., 1999). Flavopiridol, a flavonoid that is specific to cdk 1, 2 and 4, at a concentration of 1 μM and olomoucine and roscovitine, purine derivatives with specificity towards cdk 1, 2 and 5, at concentrations of 200 μM and 50 μM, respectively, protected CGNs from KCl withdrawal-induced apoptosis. This was associated with inhibition of the cdk activities, inhibition of translocation of cyclin D1, prevention of degradation of p27, and inhibition of Rb phosphorylation and degradation. Cdk4 and cyclin D as well as cdk2 and cyclin E activities are essential for Rb phosphorylation and transition of cells through G1/S checkpoint. Thus, this study suggests that upon activity withdrawal CGNs attempt to enter the cell cycle but due to the lack of an active cell cycle program this attempt is aborted and the cells take the alternative approach and undergo apoptosis. Studies in mouse neurons have also shown induction of cyclin D1 and associated kinase activity upon KCl withdrawal-induced apoptosis. This was associated with Rb hyperphosphorylation and degradation which could be inhibited by treatment with caspase inhibitors (Boutillier et al., 1999; Boutillier et al., 2000). Expression of a caspase cleavage mutant of Rb protected the cells from undergoing apoptosis thereby suggesting that physiological levels of functional Rb is necessary for survival of CGNs. This again suggests that upon lowering KCl concentrations, the neurons attempt to re-enter cell cycle but due to the absence of an active cell division cycle, they undergo apoptosis.

Since E2F1 has been implicated in apoptosis it is rational to think that E2F1 overexpression may lead to cell death. Analysis of CGNs undergoing apoptosis showed that E2F1 mRNA and protein levels were induced upon KCl withdrawal (O'Hare et al., 2000). This study also showed that adenovirus mediated overexpression of E2F1 in CGNs can induce apoptosis.

This apoptosis was p53-independent as overexpression of E2F1 in neurons from both p53+/+ and p53-/- mice showed similar levels of apoptosis. The E2F1-mediated apoptosis was found to be Bax-dependent and was associated with increased caspase 3-like activity. Studies conducted on cells from E2F1 deficient mice showed significantly higher number of surviving neurons upon withdrawal of KCl confirming that E2F1 expression is associated with enhanced apoptosis in postmitotic neurons.

Studies conducted on neurons treated with kainic acid have shown that it is associated with a transient increase in Rb phosphorylation suggesting a role for aberrant cell cycle activation (Giardina et al., 1998). When the effect of kainate treatment was compared in neurons from E2F1 deficient and E2F1 WT neurons, it was found that the neurons from E2F1 -/- mice were more resistant to KA-induced apoptosis. Thus, this study shows that excitotoxicity-induced apoptosis in neurons is also mediated through cell cycle activation, inactivation of Rb and E2F1-dependent transactivation of genes.

The above studies clearly show that activation of the components of G1 phase of cell cycle is associated with activity winthdrawal-induced apoptosis in CGNs . None of them show any evidence for entry of cells in to the S phase or expression of any of the late phase markers of cell cycle upon induction of apoptosis. It was hypothesized that the cells undergoing apoptosis acquire morphology similar to those undergoing mitosis and therefore mechanisms similar to that seen in mitotic phase of cell cycle may be activated in the apoptotic process (King and Cidlowski, 1995). This hypothesis was supported by the studies in fibroblasts where cdc2 has been shown to induce apoptosis (Yu et al., 1998). In order to determine whether cdc2 expression is associated with apoptosis in neurons, Konishi and colleagues examined CGNs undergoing activity winthdrawal-induced apoptosis (Konishi et al., 2002). Their studies showed that activity withdrawal-induced, but not growth factor withdrawal-induced, cell death in CGN is associated with induction in the G2/M kinase cdc2 (cdk1) and cdc2-mediated BAD phosphorylation. Cdc2 associates with cyclin B in the G2/M phase of cell cycle and regulates the onset of M-phase. Experiments in CGN deprived of depolarizing concentrations of KCl showed that cdc2 kinase enhanced the phosphorylation of the proapoptotic protein BAD at Ser128 residue upon apoptosis. Under normal conditions growth factor-induced phosphorylation of BAD at Ser136 leads to its sequestration by 14-3-3 proteins thus preventing it from inducing apoptosis. Under apoptotic conditions, the additional phosphorylation of BAD at Ser128 by the cdc2 kinase prevents it from getting sequestered by 14-3-3 resulting in BAD-induced apoptosis in neurons.

Cdc2 is an E2F responsive gene and induction in E2F transcriptional activity may therefore upregulate the expression of cdc2. Chromatin immunoprecipitation (ChIP) assays using E2F1 antibody and analysis of the promoter of cdc2 kinase has shown that E2F forms a complex with the promoter endogenously thereby suggesting that E2F1 can induce transactivation of cdc2 (Konishi and Bonni, 2003a). It was also shown that the expression of a dominant negative E2F1 inhibits and WT E2F1 induces cdc2 expression and apoptosis of CGN. These observations clearly show that activity withdrawal-induced apoptosis in neurons is associated with cell cycle activation, Rb phosphorylation and inactivation, and G1→S transition in CGN. It appears that the neurons may even enter the G2/M phase of cell cycle before succumbing to apoptosis. Further, the phosphorylation of BAD by cdc2 kinase reveals how cell cycle mechanisms link to the cell death machinery to bring about the apoptosis in neurons.

The cdks mentioned above are mainly exerting their effects by association with specific cyclins. For example cyclin D associates with cdks 4 and 6, cyclin E with cdk2, and cyclin A and cyclin B with cdc2. One cdk that does not depend on a cyclin to exert its activity and is mainly active in the nervous system is the cyclin dependent kinase 5 (cdk5) (Tsai et al., 1994). The regulatory subunits that activate this cdk are the p35 and p39 which are found in the neuronal tissue. P35-cdk5 complex is expressed at high levels in the adult brain and is involved in neuronal migration and axonal growth (Nikolic et al., 1996; Ohshima et al., 1999). P35 is proteolytically cleaved by calcium-dependent proteases to generate p25, which is more stable and active. The p25-cdk5 complex is hyperactive and has been shown to induce neurotoxicity (Lee et al., 2000; Patrick et al., 1999). Studies conducted using embryonic mouse brain extracts as well as bacterially expressed Rb and cdk5/p25 have shown that p25 can directly bind to Rb and induce its phosphorylation (Lee et al., 1997). In addition, studies in SY5Y cells overexpressing inducible p25 showed that it enhances phosphorylation of Rb which is blocked by roscovitine, a kinase inhibitor that inhibits cdks 1, 2 and 5 but not the cyclin D kinases cdks 4 or 6 (Hamdane et al., 2005). These findings that cdk5 can phosphorylate and inactivate Rb suggest that even in the absence of alterations in cyclins and the associated cdks, this neuronal cdk5 may induce transcriptional activation and neurodegeneration by causing inactivation of Rb.

4.2 Purkinje neurons

Extensive studies by Herrup and colleagues have shown that the different types of neurons in the cerebellum depend on each other, especially on the Purkinje neurons for trophic support and survival (Wetts and Herrup, 1982, 1983). This is termed as 'developmental dependency'. A considerably high number of cerebellar granule neuron precursor cells are generated during brain development. Studies have shown that numerical matching of the granule cells to Purkinje cells is important for normal cerebellar development and the excess number of cells that do not reach the target or that do not connect with the Purkinje cells are eliminated by apoptosis (Herrup and Sunter, 1987; Vogel et al., 1989). In the case of Purkinje neurons only a limited number of immature cells are generated which develop into the mature Purkinje cells in a cell autonomous way. Studies done in *Staggerer* and *Lurcher* mutant mice have shown that loss of Purkinje neurons is associated with loss of CGNs and inferior olive neurons (Herrup and Mullen, 1979; Rabacchi et al., 1992; Sonmez and Herrup, 1984; Vogel et al., 1991). These mutant mice show defects in the development of Purkinje neurons. In the *Staggerer* mice the Purkinje neurons never develop fully resulting in deficiency in the targets required for CGN to establish contacts. This leads to loss of neurons and these mutant mice show 100% loss of CGNs. On the other hand in the *Lurcher* mice a small percent (10%) of the CGNs survive even when 100% of the Purkinje neurons die between postnatal day 9 and 30. Analysis of CGNs and inferior olive neurons in these mice revealed that the death is associated with enhanced expression of cyclin D1, PCNA and increased DNA synthesis, as evident by BrdU incorporation (Herrup and Busser, 1995). This suggests that lack of trophic factor support induces cell cycle reentry and cell death in these neurons *in vivo*. PCNA is an S phase specific marker and this along with the induction of DNA synthesis in neurons undergoing apoptosis suggests that their death may be associated with inactivation of Rb and induction of E2F-dependent transactivation of genes. The degenerating Purkinje cells do not show any incorporation of BrdU which is indicative of a different mechanism involved in the death of these neurons in these mutant mice.

The absence of cell cycle activation in degenerating Purkinje neurons in *Staggerer* and *Lurcher* mutant mice does not mean that these cells do not re-enter cell cycle. Studies conducted in mice overexpressing the viral oncoprotein SV40 large T-antigen (T-Ag) have shown that Purkinje cell specific overexpression of T-Ag is associated with cell cycle activation and neurodegeneration (Feddersen et al., 1995; Feddersen et al., 1997). T-Ag overexpressing mice show DNA synthesis and nuclear fragmentation indicative of programmed cell death. Further, analysis of the Purkinje neurons using mutated T-Ag showed that overexpression of the Rb binding domain of this oncoprotein is sufficient to induce neurodegeneration of Purkinje neurons indicating that functional Rb is essential for the survival of these neurons.

Depending on the levels of T-Ag expression in the Purkinje cells, the mice showed variation in development of neurodegeneration and ataxia (Feddersen et al., 1997). Mice that express greater than 30 copies of the T-Ag transgene showed ataxia at 2 weeks of age. This was associated with immature Purkinje cell death and defects in cerebellar development. This suggests that normal development of Purkinje cells is essential for the proliferation, differentiation and migration of cerebellar granule cells from external to internal granule layer. Mouse with 10 copies of transgene showed ataxia at 10 weeks and those with 2 copies at 15 weeks. This study clearly shows the importance of functional Rb in terminal differentiation and protection of neurons and explains the reason for detection of high levels of Rb in the adult brain (Bernards et al., 1989; Okano et al., 1993). It has been shown that the final mitosis in Purkinje cells occurs at day 13. In mice expressing T-Ag the loss of Purkinje neurons due to cell cycle activation occurred at day 14 (2 weeks) suggesting that developing Purkinje neurons are incapable of initiating cell division.

Since E2F1 overexpression has been implicated in apoptosis, Feddersen and colleagues examined whether the levels of E2F1 is enhanced in degenerating Purkinje cells (Athanasiou et al., 1998). They found that both E2F1 and the E2F-responsive cdc2 gene were induced in the same neurons indicating the E2F-dependent transactivation of genes upon apoptosis induction. This prompted them to look at the effect of overexpression of E2F1 in Purkinje neurons. Their studies showed that overexpression of E2F1 by itself did not have any profound effect on Purkinje cell morphology or survival. But, the E2F1 overexpressing Purkinje cells showed accelerated neurodegeneration upon T-Ag overexpression suggesting that either a posttranslational modification or an association of E2F with other regulators such as dimerization partner 1 or 2 (DP1 and DP2) is necessary for induction of transactivation of genes (Athanasiou et al., 1998).

Normally, T-Ag overexpression leads to tumorigenesis in mouse tissues, including neurons of retina and CNS (al-Ubaidi et al., 1992a; al-Ubaidi et al., 1992b; Hammang et al., 1990), but in the case of Purkinje neurons it was associated with neurodegeneration, apoptois and ataxia (Feddersen et al., 1995). This suggests that T-Ag induces differential effects in different types of cells in a context specific manner, and indicates the significance of functional Rb in normal development and differentiation of the Purkinje neurons. In this context, studies in photoreceptor cells of the retina showed that if oncogene overexpression is induced prior to cessation of mitosis, it leads to tumorigenesis whereas overexpression in postmitotic cells leads to degeneration and apoptosis (al-Ubaidi et al., 1992a; al-Ubaidi et al., 1992b; Feddersen et al., 1995; Howes et al., 1994).

In vitro studies further confirmed the significance of functional Rb in survival and normal development and protection of Purkinje neurons (Padmanabhan et al., 2007). Examination of organotypic slice cultures of cerebellum taken from Sprague Dawley rats at postnatal day 4 (P4) and 9 (P9) showed a time-dependent decrease in survival of Purkinje neurons (Padmanabhan et al., 2007). It has been shown that the Purkinje neurons in slice cultures prepared from postnatal day P1 through P7 die by apoptosis (Dusart et al., 1997; Ghoumari et al., 2000). Treatment of the cultures with pharmacological inhibitors of cdks such as roscovitine, olomoucine and flavopiridol protected the neurons from undergoing apoptosis, with roscovitine showing the maximum effect (Figure 2).

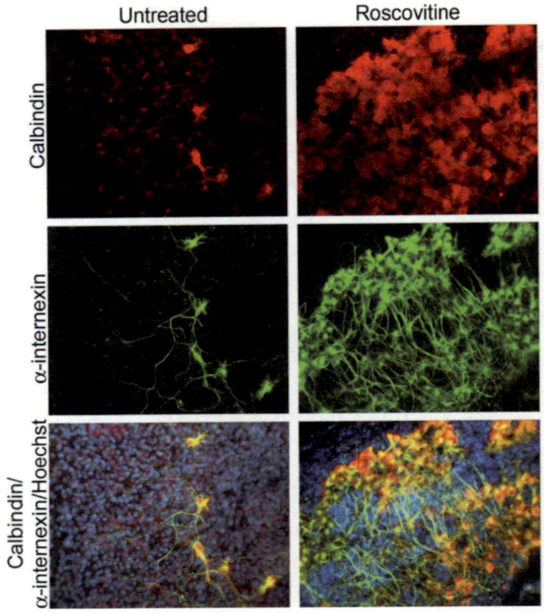

Fig. 2. Protection of Purkinje neurons by roscovitine in organotypic slice cultures: Cerebellar slice cultures from P4 rats were treated with or without 50 μM roscovitine for 1 week. Sections were fixed and stained using polyclonal calbindin (top row) and monoclonal α-internexin (middle row) antibodies. Alexa 594 fluorophore was used for detection of calbindin (red) and Alexa 488 for α-internexin (green). Hoechst was used to detect the nuclei which allowed us to view the integrity of the section. Bottom row show the composite image showing all the three staining. Sections were analyzed using a Nikon Eclipse E1000 fluorescent microscope and using Genus 2.81 software. Roscovitine protected the cell body of the neruons but not the dendrites.

Although the cdk inhibitor-treated slices showed significantly higher number of calbindin positive Purkinje neurons (Figure 2), the morphology of the cells was quite different. The elaborate dendritic arborization of the Purkinje neurons was not protected by the inhibitors; the dendritic tree showed a stunted appearance and the axons appeared to be shorter. The Purkinje neurons in the untreated sections, that survived the axotomy-induced apoptosis, showed normal dendritic arborization. This may suggest that the mechanism involved in the maintenance or protection of cell body is different from that involved in the protection of neurites. Another possibility is that the supporting cells required for normal development of Purkinje neurons are not protected by the cdk inhibitor treatment and therefore the morphology of the neurons are not maintained. Granule cells have been shown to provide the trophical support and electrical activity required for the normal development of Purkinje neurons, and Bergmann glia is necessary for the directed growth and polarity of the Purkinje dendrites. Both Purkinje cells and granule cells have been shown to express BDNF and knockout mice for BDNF show stunted growth of Purkinje neurons and loss of granule neurons (Schwartz et al., 1997). In addition, growth factors such as GDNF, NGF, NT-3, CNTF, and IGF-1 have been implicated in survival of these neurons (Segal et al., 1997). Although we tried to rescue the morphology and cell death by providing trophic support, NT3 and BDNF, we did not observe any significant protection suggesting the involvement of a more complex mechanism in the maintenance and protection of Purkinje neurons.

Analysis of the sections with the α-internexin antibody, which stains the parallel fibers of CGNs showed loss of these neurons in the slices. As discussed earlier survival of these neurons depends on the development and support from the Purkinje neurons. The fact that the cdk inhibitors were unable to protect the dendrites and axons of the Purkinje neurons suggests that this may have a profound impact on the survival of CGNs and inferior olive neurons. Normally Purkinje neurons in slices taken from rats between postnatal days P1 and P5 die within 1 week after culturing (Dusart et al., 1997). Studies with the inhibitors showed that cerebellar sections taken from P4 rats show significant protection of Purkinje neurons after 1 week in culture (Padmanabhan et al., 2007). These results clearly indicate that the Purkinje neurons in the explants undergo apoptosis through a cell cycle dependent mechanism.

Since Rb has been implicated in the survival and maintenance of differentiated state of neurons, experiments were done to determine whether Rb can protect the Purkine neurons in the organotypic slice cultures. Overexpression of a WT and phosphorylation site mutant of Rb in cerebellar sections was achieved by adenovirus-mediated method (Padmanabhan et al., 2007). Rb overexpression showed significant protection of Purkinje neurons in the slice cultures. In addition, the neurons retained their normal dendritic arbors and axons further establishing the importance of functional Rb in protection and development of normal Purkinje neurons.

5. Relevance to diseases

5.1 Cerebellar tumors

Rb plays an essential role in cell proliferation, differentiation and migration of granule cell precursors in the cerebellum. Lack of Rb during cerebellar development results in prolonged proliferation, delayed differentiation, and altered migration of precursor cells. Improper differentiation of cerebellar neurons can initiate tumors of the cerebellum (Fults, 2005). For example, one of the most common malignant tumors of the childhood is the medulloblastomas. This is a tumor of the cerebellum and it originates from transformed granule cell precursors. Sonic Hedgehog (Shh), Wingless (Wnt) and Notch signaling pathways have been implicated in proliferation, differentiation and migration of granule cells (Katoh and Katoh, 2009; Oliver et al., 2003; Wechsler-Reya and Scott, 1999). Activating mutations in Shh have been implicated in granule precursor cell proliferation and development of basal cell carcinoma and medulloblastoma. Shh-dependent cell proliferation in granule neuron precursor cells has been shown to be associated with expression of cyclins D1, D2 and E thereby promoting the cyclin-Rb pathway (Kenney and Rowitch, 2000). Granule cells in the cerebellum are generated in the external layer of cerebellum and migrate to the internal layer upon maturation. Studies in mouse models of medulloblastoma showed that granule cells in external granule layer (EGL) are involved in the development of medulloblastoma. These granule cells are immature and mitotic and when they become postmitotic, they migrate to the internal granule layer (IGL). Overexpression of Rb induced apoptosis in the cells derived from medulloblastomas implying that functional Rb is essential for the proper development, differentiation and migration of granule precursor cells. In the absence of Rb the precursor cells may continue to proliferate in the EGL layer and develop into malignant tumors.

Similar to Shh signaling, Wnt signaling has also been implicated in the development of medulloblastoma. Wnt functions through its association with the receptor Frizzled and by modulating the levels of β-catenin in the cells (Morin, 1999). When Wnt signaling is absent GSK3β phosphorylates β-catenin leading to its ubiquitination and degradation. Activation of Wnt signaling inactivates GSK3β leading to the stabilization of β-catenin. β-catenin translocates into the nucleus and transactivates LCT/TCF family of transcription factors inducing expression of genes such as c-Myc and cyclin D1 leading to aberrant cell cycle activation and cell proliferation. This also suggests that altered Wnt signaling in cerebellum can lead to activation of cyclin D-Rb axis and induction in transactivation of genes.

5.2 Ataxias

Another pathological condition that originates from defects in cerebellum is ataxia. Cerebellum plays a major role in motor coordination and movements as well as cognitive functions and damages to the cerebellum leads to loss of these functions. Studies conducted in transgenic mice with Purkinje specific expression of T-Ag showed that the oncogene expression is associated with degeneration of Purkinje neurons and developmental defects in the cerebellum (Feddersen et al., 1997). These mice developed ataxia that is characteristic of cerebellar dysfunction. T-Ag, as discussed before, associates with Rb, inhibits its binding to E2F1, and induces transactivation of genes. This suggests that cell cycle activation may play a critical role in different types of ataxia where cerebellar degeneration is a major contributor. These include Friedreich's ataxia, Ataxia Telangiectasia, congenital cerebellar ataxia etc. Loss of neuronal cell cycle control has been implicated in Ataxia-Telangiectasia, where Ataxia Telangiectasia gene is mutated (ATM), which is a neurological condition where progressive degeneration of neurons leads to major neuropathological disability (Kuljis et al., 1997; Yang and Herrup, 2005). This disease is associated with severe atrophy of the cerebellar cortical layers with extensive Purkinje and granule cell loss, dentate olivary nuclei atrophy, neuronal loss in the substantia nigra and oculomotor nuclei, spinal cord atrophy, and degenerative changes in spinal motor neurons (Crawford, 1998). The molecular mechanisms involved in the occurrence of this disease are unclear. Studies in ATM -/- mouse models have shown that vulnerable neurons in the cerebellum show ectopic expression of cell cycle proteins, which may indicate involvement of Rb and E2F (Yang and Herrup, 2005). Further studies are necessary to understand the exact molecular mechanisms involved in this and other ataxias.

6. Conclusion

In summary, *in vivo* studies conducted in mouse cerebellum from transgenic mice expressing viral oncoproteins (T-Ag), and mouse expressing neurological mutations such as *Staggerer* and *Lurcher* show that defects in development of Purkinje neurons and cerebellar granule neurons lead to abnormal development of the cerebellum and the development of ataxia. Studies with the T-Ag clearly show that the degeneration in Purkinje neurons leads to migratory defects in granule neurons and developmental defects in cerebellum. This is mainly caused by the loss of functional Rb leading to untimely cell cycle reentry of postmitotic neurons. This attempt by the postmitotic neurons to re-enter the cell cycle leads to catastrophic effects, and cells undergo apoptosis, suggesting that differentiated neurons need to be kept under tight control from re-entering the cell cycle. Once the cell cycle paradigm is activated, there is no return to the healthy state and the cells activate the apoptotic machinery to eliminate themselves. Prevention of this re-entry and maintenance of the neurons in the postmitotic state is critical for normal functioning of the brain. The *in vitro* studies in dissociated cerebellar granule neurons and organotypic slice cultures of cerebellum clearly show that both granule neurons and Purkinje neurons undergo cell cycle-mediated neurodegeneration and apoptosis (schematic, Figure 3). Although cdk inhibitors protected the neurons from undergoing apoptosis, the morphology of Purkinje neurons in the inhibitor treated cells looked abnormal. When protected by overexpression of Rb the Purkinje neurons showed very close to or normal dendritic and axonal development. This clearly suggests that the anti-apoptotic and anti-proliferative properties of Rb are essential

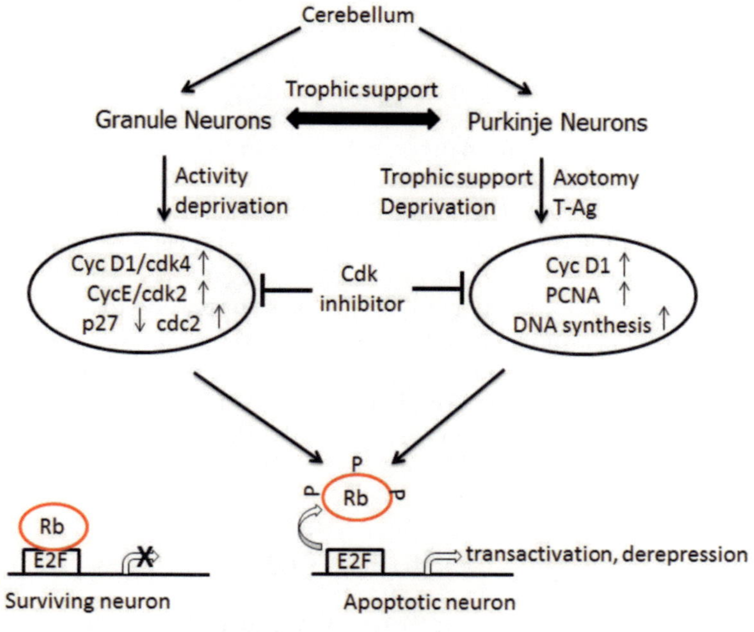

Fig. 3. Schematic showing the Rb-E2F pathway in neuronal apoptosis: Deprivation of activity or trophic facor support induces cyclins and cdks which phosphorylate Rb, release Rb from E2F and induce transactivation/derepression of E2F-dependent proapoptotic genes. Cdk inhibitors prevent activation of the kinases and protect neurons from undergoing apoptosis.

for the normal development and survival of terminally differentiated neurons. Studies using the inhibitors of cdks and overexpression of Rb suggest that maintaining functional Rb in the cerebellum is important for its normal development and functioning. These studies therefore suggest that gene therapy using Rb should be considered for therapeutic intervention of diseases of the cerebellum, such as the ataxias and medulloblastomas, where Rb inactivation and cell cycle activation are closely associated.

7. Acknowledgment

The work in JP's laboratory is supported by grants from NIH-NIA (1R21AG031429-01A2), Alzheimer's Association (IIRG-08-90842), Small Research Pilot Grant from Signature Interdisciplinary Program in Neuroscience at University of South Florida, and startup funds from the Byrd Alzheimer's Institute and Department of Molecular Medicine.

8. References

al-Ubaidi, M.R., Font, R.L., Quiambao, A.B., Keener, M.J., Liou, G.I., Overbeek, P.A., and Baehr, W. (1992a). Bilateral retinal and brain tumors in transgenic mice expressing simian virus 40 large T antigen under control of the human interphotoreceptor retinoid-binding protein promoter. J Cell Biol *119*, 1681-1687.

al-Ubaidi, M.R., Hollyfield, J.G., Overbeek, P.A., and Baehr, W. (1992b). Photoreceptor degeneration induced by the expression of simian virus 40 large tumor antigen in the retina of transgenic mice. Proc Natl Acad Sci U S A *89*, 1194-1198.

Angus, S.P., Fribourg, A.F., Markey, M.P., Williams, S.L., Horn, H.F., DeGregori, J., Kowalik, T.F., Fukasawa, K., and Knudsen, E.S. (2002). Active RB elicits late G1/S inhibition. Experimental cell research *276*, 201-213.

Ardelt, A.A., Flaris, N.A., and Roth, K.A. (1994). Neurotrophin-4 selectively promotes survival of striatal neurons in organotypic slice culture. Brain research *647*, 340-344.

Athanasiou, M.C., Yunis, W., Coleman, N., Ehlenfeldt, R., Clark, H.B., Orr, H.T., and Feddersen, R.M. (1998). The transcription factor E2F-1 in SV40 T antigen-induced cerebellar Purkinje cell degeneration. Molecular and cellular neurosciences *12*, 16-28.

Barde, Y.A. (1994). Neurotrophins: a family of proteins supporting the survival of neurons. Progress in clinical and biological research *390*, 45-56.

Barde, Y.A., Davies, A.M., Johnson, J.E., Lindsay, R.M., and Thoenen, H. (1987). Brain derived neurotrophic factor. Prog Brain Res *71*, 185-189.

Bernards, R., Shackleford, G.M., Gerber, M.R., Horowitz, J.M., Friend, S.H., Schartl, M., Bogenmann, E., Rapaport, J.M., McGee, T., Dryja, T.P., *et al.* (1989). Structure and expression of the murine retinoblastoma gene and characterization of its encoded protein. Proc Natl Acad Sci U S A *86*, 6474-6478.

Besson, A., Dowdy, S.F., and Roberts, J.M. (2008). CDK inhibitors: cell cycle regulators and beyond. Dev Cell *14*, 159-169.

Biffo, S., Dechant, G., Okazawa, H., and Barde, Y.A. (1994). Molecular control of neuronal survival in the chick embryo. Exs *71*, 39-48.

Boutillier, A.L., Kienlen-Campard, P., and Loeffler, J.P. (1999). Depolarization regulates cyclin D1 degradation and neuronal apoptosis: a hypothesis about the role of the ubiquitin/proteasome signalling pathway. The European journal of neuroscience *11*, 441-448.

Boutillier, A.L., Trinh, E., and Loeffler, J.P. (2000). Caspase-dependent cleavage of the retinoblastoma protein is an early step in neuronal apoptosis. Oncogene *19*, 2171-2178.

Burke, R.E. (1998). Programmed cell death and Parkinson's disease. Movement disorders : official journal of the Movement Disorder Society *13 Suppl 1*, 17-23.

Catterall, W.A. (2000). Structure and regulation of voltage-gated Ca2+ channels. Annual review of cell and developmental biology *16*, 521-555.

Chellappan, S., Kraus, V.B., Kroger, B., Munger, K., Howley, P.M., Phelps, W.C., and Nevins, J.R. (1992). Adenovirus E1A, simian virus 40 tumor antigen, and human papillomavirus E7 protein share the capacity to disrupt the interaction between transcription factor E2F and the retinoblastoma gene product. Proceedings of the National Academy of Sciences of the United States of America *89*, 4549-4553.

Chellappan, S.P., Hiebert, S., Mudryj, M., Horowitz, J.M., and Nevins, J.R. (1991). The E2F transcription factor is a cellular target for the RB protein. Cell *65*, 1053-1061.

Chen, P.L., Riley, D.J., and Lee, W.H. (1995). The retinoblastoma protein as a fundamental mediator of growth and differentiation signals. Critical reviews in eukaryotic gene expression *5*, 79-95.

Clarke, A.R., Maandag, E.R., van Roon, M., van der Lugt, N.M., van der Valk, M., Hooper, M.L., Berns, A., and te Riele, H. (1992). Requirement for a functional Rb-1 gene in murine development. Nature *359*, 328-330.

Cotman, C.W., and Anderson, A.J. (1995). A potential role for apoptosis in neurodegeneration and Alzheimer's disease. Molecular neurobiology *10*, 19-45.

Cotman, C.W., and Su, J.H. (1996). Mechanisms of neuronal death in Alzheimer's disease. Brain pathology *6*, 493-506.

Crawford, T.O. (1998). Ataxia telangiectasia. Semin Pediatr Neurol *5*, 287-294.

D'Mello, S.R., Borodezt, K., and Soltoff, S.P. (1997). Insulin-like growth factor and potassium depolarization maintain neuronal survival by distinct pathways: possible involvement of PI 3-kinase in IGF-1 signaling. J Neurosci *17*, 1548-1560.

D'Mello, S.R., Galli, C., Ciotti, T., and Calissano, P. (1993). Induction of apoptosis in cerebellar granule neurons by low potassium: inhibition of death by insulin-like growth factor I and cAMP. Proc Natl Acad Sci U S A *90*, 10989-10993.

D'Mello, S.R., Kuan, C.Y., Flavell, R.A., and Rakic, P. (2000). Caspase-3 is required for apoptosis-associated DNA fragmentation but not for cell death in neurons deprived of potassium. J Neurosci Res *59*, 24-31.

Dasgupta, P., Betts, V., Rastogi, S., Joshi, B., Morris, M., Brennan, B., Ordonez-Ercan, D., and Chellappan, S. (2004). Direct binding of apoptosis signal-regulating kinase 1 to retinoblastoma protein: novel links between apoptotic signaling and cell cycle machinery. The Journal of biological chemistry *279*, 38762-38769.

Dasgupta, P., Padmanabhan, J., and Chellappan, S. (2006). Rb function in the apoptosis and senescence of non-neuronal and neuronal cells: role in oncogenesis. Current molecular medicine *6*, 719-729.

de Pablo, F., Scott, L.A., and Roth, J. (1990a). Insulin and insulin-like growth factor I in early development: peptides, receptors and biological events. Endocrine reviews *11*, 558-577.

de Pablo, F., Serrano, J., Girbau, M., Alemany, J., Scavo, L., and Lesniak, M.A. (1990b). Insulin and insulin-like growth factor I action in the chick embryo: from biology to molecular endocrinology. The Journal of experimental zoology Supplement : published under auspices of the American Society of Zoologists and the Division of

Comparative Physiology and Biochemistry / the Wistar Institute of Anatomy and Biology *4*, 187-191.

Dusart, I., Airaksinen, M.S., and Sotelo, C. (1997). Purkinje cell survival and axonal regeneration are age dependent: an in vitro study. J Neurosci *17*, 3710-3726.

Farinelli, S.E., and Greene, L.A. (1996). Cell cycle blockers mimosine, ciclopirox, and deferoxamine prevent the death of PC12 cells and postmitotic sympathetic neurons after removal of trophic support. The Journal of neuroscience : the official journal of the Society for Neuroscience *16*, 1150-1162.

Feddersen, R.M., Clark, H.B., Yunis, W.S., and Orr, H.T. (1995). In vivo viability of postmitotic Purkinje neurons requires pRb family member function. Molecular and cellular neurosciences *6*, 153-167.

Feddersen, R.M., Yunis, W.S., O'Donnell, M.A., Ebner, T.J., Shen, L., Iadecola, C., Orr, H.T., and Clark, H.B. (1997). Susceptibility to cell death induced by mutant SV40 T-antigen correlates with Purkinje neuron functional development. Molecular and cellular neurosciences *9*, 42-62.

Ferrari, G., Minozzi, M.C., Toffano, G., Leon, A., and Skaper, S.D. (1989). Basic fibroblast growth factor promotes the survival and development of mesencephalic neurons in culture. Developmental biology *133*, 140-147.

Ferrer, I., Ballabriga, J., Marti, E., Perez, E., Alberch, J., and Arenas, E. (1998). BDNF up-regulates TrkB protein and prevents the death of CA1 neurons following transient forebrain ischemia. Brain pathology *8*, 253-261.

Forloni, G. (1993). beta-Amyloid neurotoxicity. Functional neurology *8*, 211-225.

Freeman, R.S., Estus, S., and Johnson, E.M., Jr. (1994). Analysis of cell cycle-related gene expression in postmitotic neurons: selective induction of Cyclin D1 during programmed cell death. Neuron *12*, 343-355.

Fults, D.W. (2005). Modeling medulloblastoma with genetically engineered mice. Neurosurg Focus *19*, E7.

Galli, C., Meucci, O., Scorziello, A., Werge, T.M., Calissano, P., and Schettini, G. (1995). Apoptosis in cerebellar granule cells is blocked by high KCl, forskolin, and IGF-1 through distinct mechanisms of action: the involvement of intracellular calcium and RNA synthesis. The Journal of neuroscience : the official journal of the Society for Neuroscience *15*, 1172-1179.

Ghoumari, A.M., Wehrle, R., Bernard, O., Sotelo, C., and Dusart, I. (2000). Implication of Bcl-2 and Caspase-3 in age-related Purkinje cell death in murine organotypic culture: an in vitro model to study apoptosis. Eur J Neurosci *12*, 2935-2949.

Giardina, S.F., Cheung, N.S., Reid, M.T., and Beart, P.M. (1998). Kainate-induced apoptosis in cultured murine cerebellar granule cells elevates expression of the cell cycle gene cyclin D1. Journal of neurochemistry *71*, 1325-1328.

Gorman, A.M., McGowan, A., O'Neill, C., and Cotter, T. (1996). Oxidative stress and apoptosis in neurodegeneration. J Neurol Sci *139 Suppl*, 45-52.

Hajimohamadreza, I., and Treherne, J.M. (1997). The role of apoptosis in neurodegenerative diseases. Progress in drug research Fortschritte der Arzneimittelforschung Progres des recherches pharmaceutiques *48*, 55-98.

Hamdane, M., Bretteville, A., Sambo, A.V., Schindowski, K., Begard, S., Delacourte, A., Bertrand, P., and Buee, L. (2005). p25/Cdk5-mediated retinoblastoma phosphorylation is an early event in neuronal cell death. J Cell Sci *118*, 1291-1298.

Hammang, J.P., Baetge, E.E., Behringer, R.R., Brinster, R.L., Palmiter, R.D., and Messing, A. (1990). Immortalized retinal neurons derived from SV40 T-antigen-induced tumors in transgenic mice. Neuron *4*, 775-782.

Hartmann, A., and Hirsch, E.C. (2001). Parkinson's disease. The apoptosis hypothesis revisited. Advances in neurology *86*, 143-153.

Herrup, K., and Busser, J.C. (1995). The induction of multiple cell cycle events precedes target-related neuronal death. Development *121*, 2385-2395.

Herrup, K., and Mullen, R.J. (1979). Staggerer chimeras: intrinsic nature of Purkinje cell defects and implications for normal cerebellar development. Brain Res *178*, 443-457.

Herrup, K., and Sunter, K. (1987). Numerical matching during cerebellar development: quantitative analysis of granule cell death in staggerer mouse chimeras. J Neurosci *7*, 829-836.

Herwig, S., and Strauss, M. (1997). The retinoblastoma protein: a master regulator of cell cycle, differentiation and apoptosis. European journal of biochemistry / FEBS *246*, 581-601.

Hiebert, S.W., Chellappan, S.P., Horowitz, J.M., and Nevins, J.R. (1992). The interaction of RB with E2F coincides with an inhibition of the transcriptional activity of E2F. Genes & development *6*, 177-185.

Hoglinger, G.U., Breunig, J.J., Depboylu, C., Rouaux, C., Michel, P.P., Alvarez-Fischer, D., Boutillier, A.L., Degregori, J., Oertel, W.H., Rakic, P., *et al.* (2007). The pRb/E2F cell-cycle pathway mediates cell death in Parkinson's disease. Proceedings of the National Academy of Sciences of the United States of America *104*, 3585-3590.

Honig, L.S., and Rosenberg, R.N. (2000). Apoptosis and neurologic disease. The American journal of medicine *108*, 317-330.

Howes, K.A., Lasudry, J.G., Albert, D.M., and Windle, J.J. (1994). Photoreceptor cell tumors in transgenic mice. Invest Ophthalmol Vis Sci *35*, 342-351.

Hume, A.J., Finkel, J.S., Kamil, J.P., Coen, D.M., Culbertson, M.R., and Kalejta, R.F. (2008). Phosphorylation of retinoblastoma protein by viral protein with cyclin-dependent kinase function. Science *320*, 797-799.

Hynes, M.A., Poulsen, K., Armanini, M., Berkemeier, L., Phillips, H., and Rosenthal, A. (1994). Neurotrophin-4/5 is a survival factor for embryonic midbrain dopaminergic neurons in enriched cultures. Journal of neuroscience research *37*, 144-154.

Irwin, M., Marin, M.C., Phillips, A.C., Seelan, R.S., Smith, D.I., Liu, W., Flores, E.R., Tsai, K.Y., Jacks, T., Vousden, K.H., *et al.* (2000). Role for the p53 homologue p73 in E2F-1-induced apoptosis. Nature *407*, 645-648.

Jacks, T., Fazeli, A., Schmitt, E.M., Bronson, R.T., Goodell, M.A., and Weinberg, R.A. (1992). Effects of an Rb mutation in the mouse. Nature *359*, 295-300.

Jacobson, M.D., Weil, M., and Raff, M.C. (1997). Programmed cell death in animal development. Cell *88*, 347-354.

Jellinger, K.A. (2001). Cell death mechanisms in neurodegeneration. Journal of cellular and molecular medicine *5*, 1-17.

Johnson, E.M., Jr. (1994). Possible role of neuronal apoptosis in Alzheimer's disease. Neurobiology of aging *15 Suppl 2*, S187-189.

Kalcheim, C., Barde, Y.A., Thoenen, H., and Le Douarin, N.M. (1987). In vivo effect of brain-derived neurotrophic factor on the survival of developing dorsal root ganglion cells. The EMBO journal *6*, 2871-2873.

Kamijo, T., Weber, J.D., Zambetti, G., Zindy, F., Roussel, M.F., and Sherr, C.J. (1998). Functional and physical interactions of the ARF tumor suppressor with p53 and

Mdm2. Proceedings of the National Academy of Sciences of the United States of America *95*, 8292-8297.

Katoh, Y., and Katoh, M. (2009). Hedgehog target genes: mechanisms of carcinogenesis induced by aberrant hedgehog signaling activation. Curr Mol Med *9*, 873-886.

Kenney, A.M., and Rowitch, D.H. (2000). Sonic hedgehog promotes G(1) cyclin expression and sustained cell cycle progression in mammalian neuronal precursors. Mol Cell Biol *20*, 9055-9067.

King, K.L., and Cidlowski, J.A. (1995). Cell cycle and apoptosis: common pathways to life and death. Journal of cellular biochemistry *58*, 175-180.

Knudsen, K.E., Booth, D., Naderi, S., Sever-Chroneos, Z., Fribourg, A.F., Hunton, I.C., Feramisco, J.R., Wang, J.Y., and Knudsen, E.S. (2000). RB-dependent S-phase response to DNA damage. Molecular and cellular biology *20*, 7751-7763.

Knusel, B., Burton, L.E., Longo, F.M., Mobley, W.C., Koliatsos, V.E., Price, D.L., and Hefti, F. (1990). Trophic actions of recombinant human nerve growth factor on cultured rat embryonic CNS cells. Experimental neurology *110*, 274-283.

Konishi, Y., and Bonni, A. (2003a). The E2F-Cdc2 cell-cycle pathway specifically mediates activity deprivation-induced apoptosis of postmitotic neurons. J Neurosci *23*, 1649-1658.

Konishi, Y., and Bonni, A. (2003b). The E2F-Cdc2 cell-cycle pathway specifically mediates activity deprivation-induced apoptosis of postmitotic neurons. The Journal of neuroscience : the official journal of the Society for Neuroscience *23*, 1649-1658.

Konishi, Y., Lehtinen, M., Donovan, N., and Bonni, A. (2002). Cdc2 phosphorylation of BAD links the cell cycle to the cell death machinery. Molecular cell *9*, 1005-1016.

Kuljis, R.O., Xu, Y., Aguila, M.C., and Baltimore, D. (1997). Degeneration of neurons, synapses, and neuropil and glial activation in a murine Atm knockout model of ataxia-telangiectasia. Proc Natl Acad Sci U S A *94*, 12688-12693.

Lee, E.Y., Chang, C.Y., Hu, N., Wang, Y.C., Lai, C.C., Herrup, K., Lee, W.H., and Bradley, A. (1992). Mice deficient for Rb are nonviable and show defects in neurogenesis and haematopoiesis. Nature *359*, 288-294.

Lee, K.Y., Helbing, C.C., Choi, K.S., Johnston, R.N., and Wang, J.H. (1997). Neuronal Cdc2-like kinase (Nclk) binds and phosphorylates the retinoblastoma protein. J Biol Chem *272*, 5622-5626.

Lee, M.S., Kwon, Y.T., Li, M., Peng, J., Friedlander, R.M., and Tsai, L.H. (2000). Neurotoxicity induces cleavage of p35 to p25 by calpain. Nature *405*, 360-364.

Lee, W.H., Chen, P.L., and Riley, D.J. (1995). Regulatory networks of the retinoblastoma protein. Annals of the New York Academy of Sciences *752*, 432-445.

Levi-Montalcini, R. (1987). The nerve growth factor: thirty-five years later. The EMBO journal *6*, 1145-1154.

Lindholm, D., Dechant, G., Heisenberg, C.P., and Thoenen, H. (1993). Brain-derived neurotrophic factor is a survival factor for cultured rat cerebellar granule neurons and protects them against glutamate-induced neurotoxicity. The European journal of neuroscience *5*, 1455-1464.

Lissy, N.A., Davis, P.K., Irwin, M., Kaelin, W.G., and Dowdy, S.F. (2000). A common E2F-1 and p73 pathway mediates cell death induced by TCR activation. Nature *407*, 642-645.

Liu, D.X., Biswas, S.C., and Greene, L.A. (2004). B-myb and C-myb play required roles in neuronal apoptosis evoked by nerve growth factor deprivation and DNA damage.

The Journal of neuroscience : the official journal of the Society for Neuroscience *24*, 8720-8725.

Liu, D.X., and Greene, L.A. (2001). Regulation of neuronal survival and death by E2F-dependent gene repression and derepression. Neuron *32*, 425-438.

Magal, E., Louis, J.C., Oudega, M., and Varon, S. (1993). CNTF promotes the survival of neonatal rat corticospinal neurons in vitro. Neuroreport *4*, 779-782.

Martin-Romero, F.J., Santiago-Josefat, B., Correa-Bordes, J., Gutierrez-Merino, C., and Fernandez-Salguero, P. (2000). Potassium-induced apoptosis in rat cerebellar granule cells involves cell-cycle blockade at the G1/S transition. Journal of molecular neuroscience : MN *15*, 155-165.

Miller, T.M., and Johnson, E.M., Jr. (1996). Metabolic and genetic analyses of apoptosis in potassium/serum-deprived rat cerebellar granule cells. The Journal of neuroscience : the official journal of the Society for Neuroscience *16*, 7487-7495.

Morin, P.J. (1999). beta-catenin signaling and cancer. Bioessays *21*, 1021-1030.

Nath, N., Wang, S., Betts, V., Knudsen, E., and Chellappan, S. (2003). Apoptotic and mitogenic stimuli inactivate Rb by differential utilization of p38 and cyclin-dependent kinases. Oncogene *22*, 5986-5994.

Nevins, J.R., Chellappan, S.P., Mudryj, M., Hiebert, S., Devoto, S., Horowitz, J., Hunter, T., and Pines, J. (1991). E2F transcription factor is a target for the RB protein and the cyclin A protein. Cold Spring Harbor symposia on quantitative biology *56*, 157-162.

Nikolic, M., Dudek, H., Kwon, Y.T., Ramos, Y.F., and Tsai, L.H. (1996). The cdk5/p35 kinase is essential for neurite outgrowth during neuronal differentiation. Genes Dev *10*, 816-825.

O'Hare, M.J., Hou, S.T., Morris, E.J., Cregan, S.P., Xu, Q., Slack, R.S., and Park, D.S. (2000). Induction and modulation of cerebellar granule neuron death by E2F-1. The Journal of biological chemistry *275*, 25358-25364.

Ohshima, T., Gilmore, E.C., Longenecker, G., Jacobowitz, D.M., Brady, R.O., Herrup, K., and Kulkarni, A.B. (1999). Migration defects of cdk5(-/-) neurons in the developing cerebellum is cell autonomous. J Neurosci *19*, 6017-6026.

Okano, H.J., Pfaff, D.W., and Gibbs, R.B. (1993). RB and Cdc2 expression in brain: correlations with 3H-thymidine incorporation and neurogenesis. J Neurosci *13*, 2930-2938.

Oliver, T.G., Grasfeder, L.L., Carroll, A.L., Kaiser, C., Gillingham, C.L., Lin, S.M., Wickramasinghe, R., Scott, M.P., and Wechsler-Reya, R.J. (2003). Transcriptional profiling of the Sonic hedgehog response: a critical role for N-myc in proliferation of neuronal precursors. Proceedings of the National Academy of Sciences of the United States of America *100*, 7331-7336.

Oppenheim, R.W. (1991). Cell death during development of the nervous system. Annu Rev Neurosci *14*, 453-501.

Padmanabhan, J., Brown, K., and Shelanski, M.L. (2007). Cell cycle inhibition and retinoblastoma protein overexpression prevent Purkinje cell death in organotypic slice cultures. Developmental neurobiology *67*, 818-826.

Padmanabhan, J., Park, D.S., Greene, L.A., and Shelanski, M.L. (1999). Role of cell cycle regulatory proteins in cerebellar granule neuron apoptosis. The Journal of neuroscience : the official journal of the Society for Neuroscience *19*, 8747-8756.

Park, D.S., Levine, B., Ferrari, G., and Greene, L.A. (1997a). Cyclin dependent kinase inhibitors and dominant negative cyclin dependent kinase 4 and 6 promote survival of NGF-deprived sympathetic neurons. The Journal of neuroscience : the official journal of the Society for Neuroscience *17*, 8975-8983.

Park, D.S., Morris, E.J., Greene, L.A., and Geller, H.M. (1997b). G1/S cell cycle blockers and inhibitors of cyclin-dependent kinases suppress camptothecin-induced neuronal apoptosis. The Journal of neuroscience : the official journal of the Society for Neuroscience *17*, 1256-1270.

Park, D.S., Morris, E.J., Padmanabhan, J., Shelanski, M.L., Geller, H.M., and Greene, L.A. (1998a). Cyclin-dependent kinases participate in death of neurons evoked by DNA-damaging agents. The Journal of cell biology *143*, 457-467.

Park, D.S., Morris, E.J., Stefanis, L., Troy, C.M., Shelanski, M.L., Geller, H.M., and Greene, L.A. (1998b). Multiple pathways of neuronal death induced by DNA-damaging agents, NGF deprivation, and oxidative stress. The Journal of neuroscience : the official journal of the Society for Neuroscience *18*, 830-840.

Patrick, G.N., Zukerberg, L., Nikolic, M., de la Monte, S., Dikkes, P., and Tsai, L.H. (1999). Conversion of p35 to p25 deregulates Cdk5 activity and promotes neurodegeneration. Nature *402*, 615-622.

Pomerantz, J., Schreiber-Agus, N., Liegeois, N.J., Silverman, A., Alland, L., Chin, L., Potes, J., Chen, K., Orlow, I., Lee, H.W., *et al.* (1998). The Ink4a tumor suppressor gene product, p19Arf, interacts with MDM2 and neutralizes MDM2's inhibition of p53. Cell *92*, 713-723.

Rabacchi, S.A., Bailly, Y., Delhaye-Bouchaud, N., Herrup, K., and Mariani, J. (1992). Role of the target in synapse elimination: studies in cerebellum of developing lurcher mutants and adult chimeric mice. J Neurosci *12*, 4712-4720.

Rabacchi, S.A., Kruk, B., Hamilton, J., Carney, C., Hoffman, J.R., Meyer, S.L., Springer, J.E., and Baird, D.H. (1999). BDNF and NT4/5 promote survival and neurite outgrowth of pontocerebellar mossy fiber neurons. Journal of neurobiology *40*, 254-269.

Raff, M.C. (1992). Social controls on cell survival and cell death. Nature *356*, 397-400.

Raff, M.C., Barres, B.A., Burne, J.F., Coles, H.S., Ishizaki, Y., and Jacobson, M.D. (1993). Programmed cell death and the control of cell survival: lessons from the nervous system. Science *262*, 695-700.

Rakowicz, W.P., Staples, C.S., Milbrandt, J., Brunstrom, J.E., and Johnson, E.M., Jr. (2002). Glial cell line-derived neurotrophic factor promotes the survival of early postnatal spinal motor neurons in the lateral and medial motor columns in slice culture. The Journal of neuroscience : the official journal of the Society for Neuroscience *22*, 3953-3962.

Riley, D.J., Lee, E.Y., and Lee, W.H. (1994). The retinoblastoma protein: more than a tumor suppressor. Annual review of cell biology *10*, 1-29.

Sakai, K., Suzuki, K., Tanaka, S., and Koike, T. (1999). Up-regulation of cyclin D1 occurs in apoptosis of immature but not mature cerebellar granule neurons in culture. Journal of neuroscience research *58*, 396-406.

Savitz, S.I., and Rosenbaum, D.M. (1998). Apoptosis in neurological disease. Neurosurgery *42*, 555-572; discussion 573-554.

Schwartz, P.M., Borghesani, P.R., Levy, R.L., Pomeroy, S.L., and Segal, R.A. (1997). Abnormal cerebellar development and foliation in BDNF-/- mice reveals a role for neurotrophins in CNS patterning. Neuron *19*, 269-281.

Segal, R.A., Rua, L., and Schwartz, P. (1997). Neurotrophins and programmed cell death during cerebellar development. Adv Neurol *72*, 79-86.

Serrano, J., Shuldiner, A.R., Roberts, C.T., Jr., LeRoith, D., and de Pablo, F. (1990). The insulin-like growth factor I (IGF-I) gene is expressed in chick embryos during early organogenesis. Endocrinology *127*, 1547-1549.

Sonmez, E., and Herrup, K. (1984). Role of staggerer gene in determining cell number in cerebellar cortex. II. Granule cell death and persistence of the external granule cell layer in young mouse chimeras. Brain Res *314*, 271-283.

Stefanis, L., Park, D.S., Friedman, W.J., and Greene, L.A. (1999). Caspase-dependent and -independent death of camptothecin-treated embryonic cortical neurons. The Journal of neuroscience : the official journal of the Society for Neuroscience *19*, 6235-6247.

Stefanis, L., Troy, C.M., Qi, H., Shelanski, M.L., and Greene, L.A. (1998). Caspase-2 (Nedd-2) processing and death of trophic factor-deprived PC12 cells and sympathetic neurons occur independently of caspase-3 (CPP32)-like activity. The Journal of neuroscience : the official journal of the Society for Neuroscience *18*, 9204-9215.

Stevaux, O., and Dyson, N.J. (2002). A revised picture of the E2F transcriptional network and RB function. Current opinion in cell biology *14*, 684-691.

Tao, W., and Levine, A.J. (1999). P19(ARF) stabilizes p53 by blocking nucleo-cytoplasmic shuttling of Mdm2. Proceedings of the National Academy of Sciences of the United States of America *96*, 6937-6941.

Troy, C.M., Rabacchi, S.A., Friedman, W.J., Frappier, T.F., Brown, K., and Shelanski, M.L. (2000). Caspase-2 mediates neuronal cell death induced by beta-amyloid. The Journal of neuroscience : the official journal of the Society for Neuroscience *20*, 1386-1392.

Troy, C.M., Rabacchi, S.A., Hohl, J.B., Angelastro, J.M., Greene, L.A., and Shelanski, M.L. (2001). Death in the balance: alternative participation of the caspase-2 and -9 pathways in neuronal death induced by nerve growth factor deprivation. The Journal of neuroscience : the official journal of the Society for Neuroscience *21*, 5007-5016.

Troy, C.M., Stefanis, L., Greene, L.A., and Shelanski, M.L. (1997). Nedd2 is required for apoptosis after trophic factor withdrawal, but not superoxide dismutase (SOD1) downregulation, in sympathetic neurons and PC12 cells. The Journal of neuroscience : the official journal of the Society for Neuroscience *17*, 1911-1918.

Troy, C.M., Stefanis, L., Prochiantz, A., Greene, L.A., and Shelanski, M.L. (1996). The contrasting roles of ICE family proteases and interleukin-1beta in apoptosis induced by trophic factor withdrawal and by copper/zinc superoxide dismutase down-regulation. Proceedings of the National Academy of Sciences of the United States of America *93*, 5635-5640.

Tsai, L.H., Delalle, I., Caviness, V.S., Jr., Chae, T., and Harlow, E. (1994). p35 is a neural-specific regulatory subunit of cyclin-dependent kinase 5. Nature *371*, 419-423.

Tuttle, J.B., Mackey, T., and Steers, W.D. (1994). NGF, bFGF and CNTF increase survival of major pelvic ganglion neurons cultured from the adult rat. Neuroscience letters *173*, 94-98.

Vogel, M.W., McInnes, M., Zanjani, H.S., and Herrup, K. (1991). Cerebellar Purkinje cells provide target support over a limited spatial range: evidence from lurcher chimeric mice. Brain Res Dev Brain Res *64*, 87-94.

Vogel, M.W., Sunter, K., and Herrup, K. (1989). Numerical matching between granule and Purkinje cells in lurcher chimeric mice: a hypothesis for the trophic rescue of granule cells from target-related cell death. J Neurosci *9*, 3454-3462.

Wang, J.Y. (1997). Retinoblastoma protein in growth suppression and death protection. Current opinion in genetics & development *7*, 39-45.

Wang, J.Y., Knudsen, E.S., and Welch, P.J. (1994). The retinoblastoma tumor suppressor protein. Advances in cancer research *64*, 25-85.

Wang, S., Nath, N., Fusaro, G., and Chellappan, S. (1999a). Rb and prohibitin target distinct regions of E2F1 for repression and respond to different upstream signals. Molecular and cellular biology *19*, 7447-7460.

Wang, S., Nath, N., Minden, A., and Chellappan, S. (1999b). Regulation of Rb and E2F by signal transduction cascades: divergent effects of JNK1 and p38 kinases. The EMBO journal *18*, 1559-1570.

Weber, J.D., Jeffers, J.R., Rehg, J.E., Randle, D.H., Lozano, G., Roussel, M.F., Sherr, C.J., and Zambetti, G.P. (2000). p53-independent functions of the p19(ARF) tumor suppressor. Genes & development *14*, 2358-2365.

Wechsler-Reya, R., and Scott, M.P. (2001). The developmental biology of brain tumors. Annual review of neuroscience *24*, 385-428.

Wechsler-Reya, R.J., and Scott, M.P. (1999). Control of neuronal precursor proliferation in the cerebellum by Sonic Hedgehog. Neuron *22*, 103-114.

Weinberg, R.A. (1989a). Positive and negative controls on cell growth. Biochemistry *28*, 8263-8269.

Weinberg, R.A. (1989b). The Rb gene and the negative regulation of cell growth. Blood *74*, 529-532.

Weinberg, R.A. (1990). The retinoblastoma gene and cell growth control. Trends in biochemical sciences *15*, 199-202.

Weinberg, R.A. (1991). Tumor suppressor genes. Science *254*, 1138-1146.

Weinberg, R.A. (1995). The retinoblastoma protein and cell cycle control. Cell *81*, 323-330.

Wetts, R., and Herrup, K. (1982). Interaction of granule, Purkinje and inferior olivary neurons in lurcher chimeric mice. II. Granule cell death. Brain Res *250*, 358-362.

Wetts, R., and Herrup, K. (1983). Direct correlation between Purkinje and granule cell number in the cerebella of lurcher chimeras and wild-type mice. Brain Res *312*, 41-47.

Yanagisawa, K. (2000). Neuronal death in Alzheimer's disease. Internal medicine *39*, 328-330.

Yang, Y., and Herrup, K. (2005). Loss of neuronal cell cycle control in ataxia-telangiectasia: a unified disease mechanism. J Neurosci *25*, 2522-2529.

Yu, D., Jing, T., Liu, B., Yao, J., Tan, M., McDonnell, T.J., and Hung, M.C. (1998). Overexpression of ErbB2 blocks Taxol-induced apoptosis by upregulation of p21Cip1, which inhibits p34Cdc2 kinase. Mol Cell *2*, 581-591.

Yuan, J., and Yankner, B.A. (2000). Apoptosis in the nervous system. Nature *407*, 802-809.

Zaika, A., Irwin, M., Sansome, C., and Moll, U.M. (2001). Oncogenes induce and activate endogenous p73 protein. The Journal of biological chemistry *276*, 11310-11316.

Zhang, C., Brandemihl, A., Lau, D., Lawton, A., and Oakley, B. (1997). BDNF is required for the normal development of taste neurons in vivo. Neuroreport *8*, 1013-1017.

Zhang, Y., Xiong, Y., and Yarbrough, W.G. (1998). ARF promotes MDM2 degradation and stabilizes p53: ARF-INK4a locus deletion impairs both the Rb and p53 tumor suppression pathways. Cell *92*, 725-734.

8

Cytoskeletal Organization and Rb Tumor Suppressor Gene

Yi-Jang Lee[1,*], Pei-Hsun Chiang[1] and Peter C. Keng[2]
[1]*Department of Biomedical Imaging and Radiological Sciences, National Yang-Ming University, Taipei*
[2]*Cancer Center, School of Medicine and Dentistry, University of Rochester, Rochester, NY*
[1]*Taiwan, R.O.C.*
[2]*USA*

1. Introduction

Cell cycle progression is dependent on a series of molecular regulation after cells are stimulated by growth factors. Growth factors bind to corresponding surface receptors and relay the signals through protein phosphorylation to trigger gene expression. Phosphorylation of retinoblastoma protein (Rb) is to release E2F family of transcription factors for DNA replication. In adherent cells, the actin filament plays an important role for anchorage, locomotion, morphological maintenance, and cell division (1). These mechanical characteristics influence cell cycle progression, and mediate cells responding to extracellular stimulations. The cyclin-dependent kinases (CDKs) are responsible for cell cycle transition through different phases. For G1 phase progression, the G1 cyclins associated CDKs can phosphorylate and inactivate Rb. Because the phosphorylation sites of Rb are multiple, they become a family of checkpoint to prevent release of E2F transcription factor under a stress condition, such as DNA damage. In addition, the CDKs activity and Rb phosphorylation are ablated by the family of CDK inhibitors (CKIs), including INK4 and CIP/KIP family proteins (2). The underlying mechanisms by which the intact actin filaments regulated cell cycle progression have been reviewed in literatures, although the pathways are diverse from different research results. However, it appears that Rb activity is commonly affected by destabilizing the actin cytoskeleton. Therefore, it is believed that growth factor stimulated actin cytoskeletal organization can regulate Rb activity for G1 phase progression and DNA replication.

Although actin cytoskeletal organization affects Rb activity, the cell cycle regulatory components have been recently reported to influence actin organization and cell motility (3). It is largely associated with CIP/KIP family proteins when they relocate to cytoplasm from nucleus. They inhibit Rho small GTPase family protein for actin architectures formation. Interestingly, Rb may regulate CIP/KIP protein expression through E2F transcriptional activity (4), and this observation implies that an autoregulatory mechanism may exist

* Corresponding Author

between actin cytoskeletal organization and Rb for regulating cell growth and cell cycle progression. Investigation of these biological events would contribute to cancer research and therapeutic design for cancer treatment or prevention.

2. Actin cytoskeletal reorganization during cell cycle progression

The cytoskeleton consists of three different types of cytosolic fibers that include actin filaments (also named microfilaments), intermediate filaments, and microtubule. Of the three types of fibers, actin filaments are primarily responsible for cell mobility, anchorage, and shape maintenance. Actin filaments are formed by polymerizing the ATP-bound actin subunits, so called G-actin, through a energy-required dynamic process. Actin filaments can be organized into different types of actin cytoskeletons including stress fibers, lamellipodia, and filapodia distributed in different regions of cells for specific functions. It is well-known that Rho small GTPase family proteins are responsible for actin organization. Organization of actin filaments is associated with cell growth depending on cell adhesion and mitogenic stimulation (5).

Accumulated evidences have supported the essence of actin cytoskeleton for cell division and proliferation. In fibroblasts, addition of growth factors or other mitogenic stimulation can promote the generation and reorganization of actin cytoskeleton through the small G proteins, including Rac, Cdc42, and Rho (6). Rac and Cdc42 are important for formation of lamellipodia and filapodia at the leading edges of cells, while Rho is responsible for formation of stress fibers. Actin filaments are organized into different types of actin structures to support cell growth after mitogenic stimulation. Moreover, actin filaments are organized at the focal contacts, in which integrins and other cytoskeletal proteins are present for cell attachment (7). Formation of focal contacts is important for activating a series of signaling pathways such as phosphatidylinositol 3-kinase (PI3-kinase) and mitogen-activated protein kinase (MAPK) pathways (8, 9). Actin filaments are important for transducing signals from extracellular matrix into cells for growth. Inhibition of actin filaments after cell attachment leads to blockage of signaling pathways and subsequent growth arrest (10-12). Actin filaments and cell adhesion are also important for cell cycle progression (13). It has been reported that cells with disorganized actin architecture are unable to initiate DNA synthesis (14). Therefore, it appears that actin filaments are important for cell growth and normal cell cycle progression.

Actin filaments are also important for cell division at the telophase during mitosis. Myosin II, one of the actin-binding proteins that moves on actin filaments, binds to actin filaments to form the contractile ring at the middle part of the dividing cell and to pull the plasma membrane inward to form a cleavage furrow (15). Disruption of actin filaments at cytokinesis can lead to failure of division and growth arrest. Collectively, organization of actin filaments is associated with cell growth in both cell signaling and structural aspects.

The distribution of actin cytoskeleton in different phase of the cell cycle has been studied more than two decades. Mitotic phase is the most obvious dynamic stage that microtubule and actin cytoskeletal reorganization can be detected. It is broadly accepted that microtubule formed spindles are critical for chromosomal segregation during mitosis. These fine-tune mitotic spindles are then required for driving the cytokinesis, a cell dividing step ablated by the actin filaments and myosin II sliding machine, for separation of the daughter cells (16-18). On the other hand, the role of actin filaments on spindle assembly and positioning are less studied. In fact, the theories of actin cytoskeletal formation in mitotic phase are debated. Investigation of actin cytoskeletal organization in higher plant cells such as meristematic root-tip cells of Allium and staminal hairs have shown that the cytoplasmic actin filaments cannot be detected until the entry of cytokinesis (19-21). The last moment for visualizing the actin filaments right before cells entering the mitosis is likely to be the preprophase (22). Reorganization of actin filaments is found at the contractile ring accompanied by the formation of cleavage furrow, while disruption of actin reorganization using cytochalasin leads to mitotic arrest and aneuploid formation (23-25). However, accumulated literatures also demonstrate that actin filaments dramatically influence the mitotic spindle positioning and assembly not only in plant cells but also in fruitflies, C. elegans zygotes, Xenopus embryos and mouse oocytes during syncytial divisions (26-33). The role of actin filaments is to regulate astral microtubule growth and spindle migration by reorganizing in the cortical region (34). Disruption of cortical actin filaments leads to misorientation of spindles and cell cycle arrest (35). Also, myosin-10 and actin filaments play cooperative but distinct functions on the mitotic spindle formation, proper spindle anchoring, spindle pole integrity, spindle length control, and mitotic progression. We looked into the different stages of anaphase and showed that actin cytoskeletal organization also changed and orchestrated with microtubule for cell division (Figure 1). Taken together, it has become clear that the actin cytoskeleton can interact with microtubule organized spindle fibers for mitotic progression and cell divisions.

Although actin cytoskeletal organization has been well-studied in the mitotic phase, the shape variations of actin cytoskeleton in the interphase remain unclear. The interphase of cell cycle includes G1, S and G2 phase. However, the actin organization in each phase is not well described in the literature. Yu et al. investigated the actin dynamics during the cell cycle in suspension-cultured tobacco BY-2 (*Nicotiana tabacum* L. cv Bright Yellow) cells using a green fluorescent protein (GFP) fused mouse Talin (mTalin) gene, which can indicate the positions of actin cytoskeleton in the plant cells. Their results clearly indicate the positions of cortical actin cytoskeletal networks in the interphase, and they are altered organized and even disappeared before cells enter mitosis and pre-prophase. Instead, the actin cytoskeletons relocalize to the future equatorial plane and centrally located nucleus and vesicles. Therefore, it is believed that actin cytoskeletal organization should vary in different stages of interphase. We have synchronized human non-small lung cancer H1299 cells at G1/S phase boundary using the double thymidine block protocol, and collected cells at different time intervals for staining of actin cytoskeletal organization using the fluorescine-conjugated phalloidin. As shown in figure 2, the actin networks concentrated around nucleus during S phase and pre-prophase (Figure 2). The cortical actin cytoskeleton formed in mitotic phase are consistent with the results reported previously (36), while the actin assemblies are also visualized between segregating chromosomes from the early anaphase to telophase. Actins are organized to visible stress fibers in the G1 phase and mediate morphological maintenance and spreading. The actin architectures are also continuously changed in the G1 phase progression. Although the underlying mechanisms remain to be studied for the association between cell cycle and actin cytoskeletal organization, we have found that the level of actin depolymerizing factor cofilin-1, a protein required for actin dynamics and reorganization, is also changed in G1 to S phase progression (unpublished data). The activity of cofilin-1 has been reported to be essential for G2/M phase progression

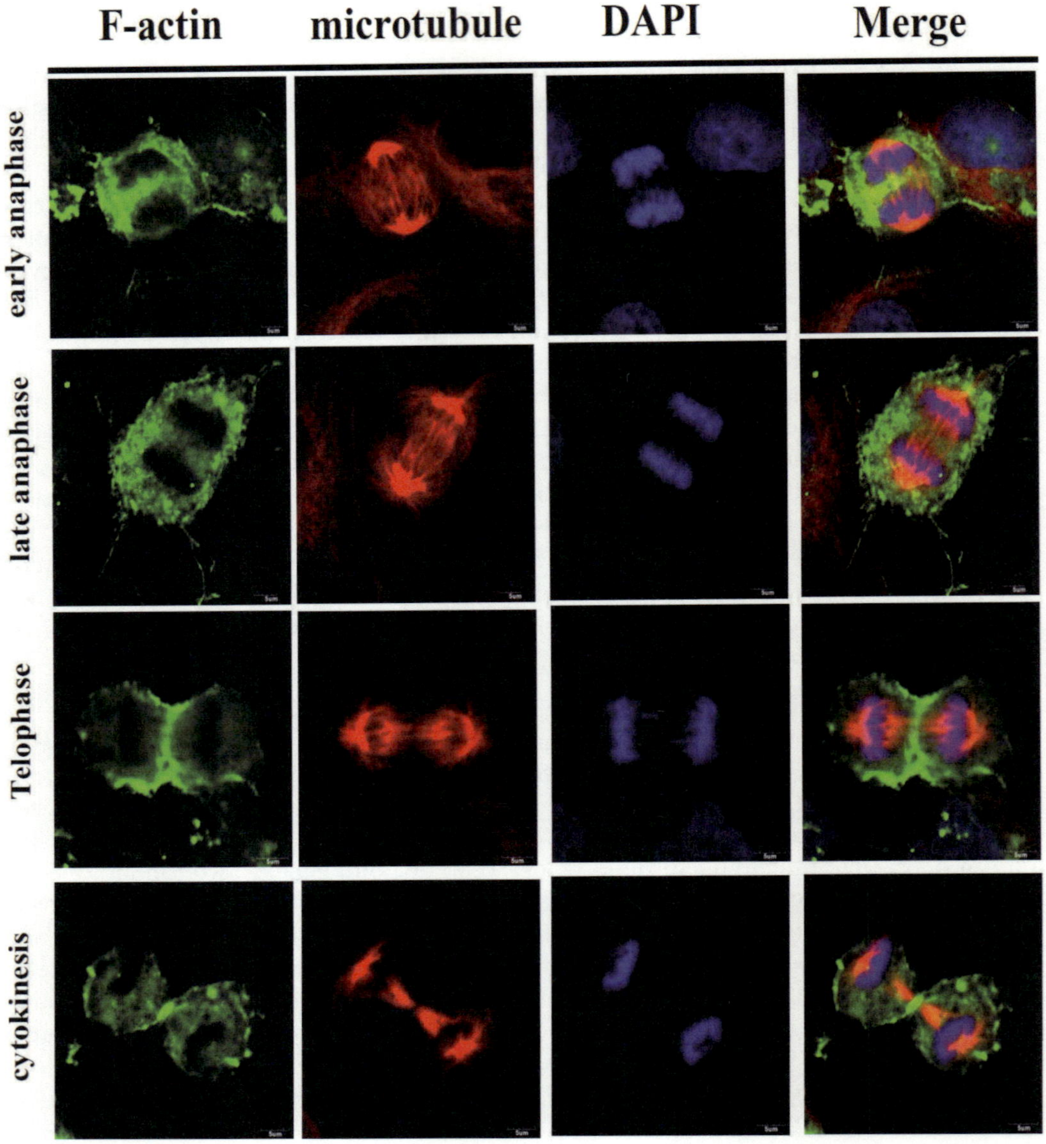

Lee YJ et al.

Fig. 1. Coordination of actin filaments and microtubules for mitotic cells passing from anaphase to telophase and cytokinesis in human non-small lung cancer H1299 cells. The conventional fiber-like structures were not visualized, while the cortical actin cytoskeletons are formed. F-actin was stained by fluorescine-conjugated phalloidin; microtubule was stained by anti-tubulin antibody; DAPI (4',6-diamidino-2-phenylindole) was used for nuclear staining.

(37, 38). We have also found that over-expression of cofilin-1 can inhibit G1 phase progression (39, 40). Thus, cofilin-1 may regulate actin cytoskeleton not only in the G2/M phase but also in G1 and S phase progression.

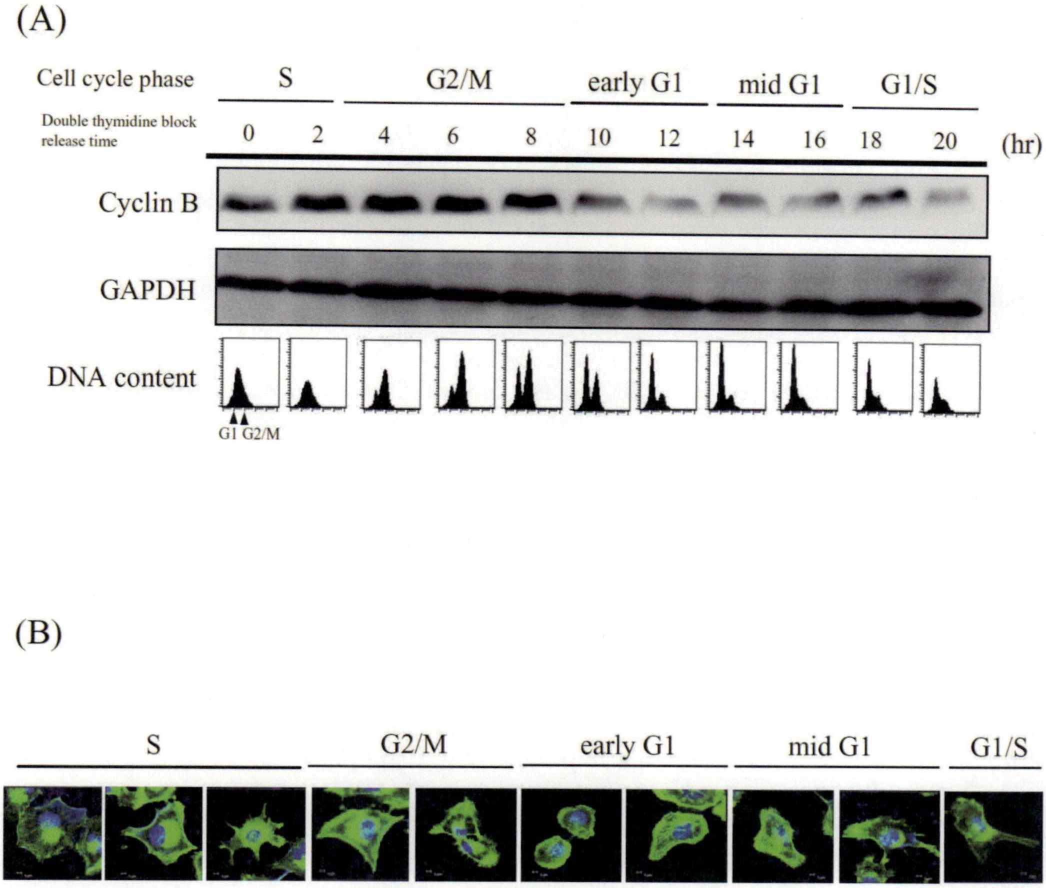

Lee YJ et al.

Fig. 2. The change of actin architectures during cell cycle progression. H1299 cells were synchronized in S phase using double thymidine block. (A) The cell cycle progression from S phase to next G1/S boundary was demonstrated by DNA histogram and the expression of cyclin B; (B) cells were collected at different stage of the cell cycle and stained for actin cytoskeleton using fluorescine-conjugated phalloidin.

3. Molecular events for cell cycle progression in mammalian cells

In eucaryotes, cell proliferation is partially dependent on cell cycle progression. Cyclin and cyclin-dependent kinases (CDK) are required for progression through gap phases (G1 and G2), DNA replication (S), and chromosome segregation (M) phases of the cell cycle. Protein complexes of cyclin and cyclin-dependent kinase (CDK) can phosphorylate specific downstream substrates, including retinoblastoma tumor suppressor protein (Rb) or anaphase-promoting complex (APC), for G1/S or M phase transition, respectively (41, 42). The activity of cyclin/CDK for G1 phase progression is regulated by CDK inhibitors, which can bind to cyclin/CDK and inhibit its activity. On the other hand, the CDK inhibitors $p21^{CIP1}$ and $p27^{KIP1}$ are indispensible for cyclin/CDK activity, suggesting that a stoichiometric balance is existed among cyclins, CDKs and CDK inhibitors (2, 43). Also, cell cycle progression can be inhibited by genotoxic stresses, such as ionizing radiation and some chemotherapeutic agents. In normal cells, activation of tumor suppressor gene p53 is usually involved in this type of response.

Different types of cyclins (A, B, C, D, and E) and CDKs (1, 2, 3, 4, and 6) are responsible for the progression of cells into different stages of cell cycle. Cyclin A binds to CDK2 for S-G2 phase progression, while cyclin B binds to CDK1 for entry into M phase. The cyclin C/CDK3 complex can promote Rb-dependent G0 phase exit (44). Cyclin D binds to CDK4/6 and cyclin E binds to CDK2 for G1 phase progression, although the latter is primarily responsible for late G1 phase or G1-S phase transition. Cyclin D consists of three closely related D-type cyclins, named Cyclin D1, D2, and D3. Expression of different types of cyclin D for G1 phase progression is likely to be tissue-specific (45). For G1 to S phase progression, Rb is phosphorylated by cyclin D-CDK4/6 and cyclin E-CDK2 to release E2F1, an important transcription factor belonging to the E2F protein family for entry into S phase (46-49). The gene targets of E2F1 are versatile and involved in DNA synthesis and G1/S progression, including DNA polymerase alpha, cyclin E, and E2F1 itself (50, 51).

Rb is a phosphoprotein containing sixteen serine/theronine sites that can be recognized by cyclin/CDKs. Mutations of nine of these consensus phosphorylation sites, including seven sites at the C-terminal and two sites at the insert region of Rb, are sufficient to constitutively active Rb and block DNA replication (52-54). Also, mutations of this phosphorylation site can cause different cell cycle and apoptotic effects in Rat-16 cells exposed to various stimuli, such as tumor necrosis factor, doxorubicin or staurosporine (55). In addition, Rb may mediate DNA damage response (DDR). It has been reported that Rb-deficient cells are incapable of cell cycle arrest and are hypersensitive to apoptosis following DNA damage (56). This result suggests that Rb may protect cells from DNA damage-induced apoptosis. However, phosphorylation of Rb via p38 kinase or ASK1 can inactivate Rb and promote apoptosis (57-60). These apoptosis-associated phosphorylation sites are independent of those targeted by cyclin/CDKs on Rb (60).

Although Rb phosphorylation is mainly mediated by D cyclin-CDK4/6 and E cyclin-CDK2 in the G1 phase, high dose of ionizing radiation induced DNA damage can permanently cause G2 phase arrest accompanied by a gradual accumulated hypophosphorylated Rb (61). Because cyclin B-CDK1 is responsible for G2 phase progression, reduced CDK1 activity is likely to be the cause of hypophosphorylated Rb in G2 phase. Interestingly, CDK1 has been reported to be the only essential cell cycle CDK because it can bind to all cyclins and control the Rb phosphorylation (62). Although it is difficult to demonstrate that cyclin B-CDK1 can mediate Rb phosphorylation in the G1 phase, it is plausible that Rb phosphorylation is ablated by CDK1 in the G2 phase. Actually, Rb phosphorylation is accompanied by the expression of cyclin B during mitosis. That is, Rb phosphorylation and cyclin B are concomitantly decreased from the prophase to telophase of mitosis (63). Besides, it has been reported that phosphorylation of amino terminus of Rb protein is mediated by a G2/M phase specific cell cycle-regulated Rb/histone H1 kinase (RbK), a kinase exhibits different enzymatic activity compared to CDK1 and CDK2 (64, 65). RbK may play a role in G2 checkpoint by controlling the Rb activity. Taken together, phosphorylation of Rb protein is important for cell cycle checkpoint at different phases.

Rb was the first identified tumor suppressor gene. Rb protein family members include Rb, p130, and p107 genes (66). However, Rb is the only most frequent mutated or deleted gene in different types of human cancers (48, 67). The functions of Rb are to sequester E2F family of transcription factors and other proteins associated with apoptosis, DNA damage response, differentiation, protein kinases, hormone regulation, and so on (68-72). Inactivation of Rb can be approached by optimal phosphorylation on the Rb protein, or by viral oncoproteins such as E7 protein of human papilloma virus, adenovirus E1A and SV40 large T-antigen that can occupy the pocket domain of Rb (48, 60, 73). The extracellular growth factors can bind to the surface receptors and activate ras/raf/mitogenic activated protein kinase (MAPK) cascade, which promote G1 phase progression by activate cyclin D-CDK4/6 and cyclinE/A-CDK2 activity. Phosphorylation of Rb by these CDKs not only releases E2F transcription factor but also remodels the chromatin structures by escaping from the repressive functions mediated by histone deacetylation complex (HDAC) and BRG1/BRM ATPase, the human homolog of yeast SWI2/SNF2 chromatin remodeling factors (60, 74-76). Mutation or over-expression of surface receptors may over-activate intracellular Ras or myc pathway that constitutively inactivates Rb for accelerating the G1/S phase progression and leads to tumorigenesis (77). Alternatively, mutation or inactivation of CDK inhibitors may also lead to excessive inactivation of Rb even the mitogenic signaling pathway is normally regulated. The role of CDK inhibitors on regulation of cell cycle and Rb activity is discussed next.

4. Regulation of cyclin/CDK on Rb inactivation by CDK inhibitors

The kinase activities of cyclin D-CDK4/6 and cyclin E-CDK2 are required for cells to progress through the G1 phase. Regulation of CDK activity is dependent on the amount of CDK inhibitors (CKIs) in cells. While the basal level of CKI is required for the formation of cyclin/CDK complex and the maintenance of its activity, a high level of CKI tends to inhibit cyclin/CDK activity (78-81). The physical interactions between CKI and cyclin/CDK is required to stabilize or inhibit the activities of CDKs.

Two families of CKIs have been discovered for controlling the activity of cyclin/CDK. One of the families is INK4, which is named for its ability of an inhibition of CDK4 activity. Members of this family are $p16^{INK4a}$, $p15^{INK4b}$, $p18^{INK4c}$, and $p19^{INK4d}$ and they specifically bind to CDK4,or CDK6, but not other CDKs. Members of CIP/KIP family containing broader spectrum inhibition of CDK2 and CDK4/6. This family includes $p21^{CIP1}$, $p27^{KIP1}$, and $p57^{kip2}$, and they can bind to both cyclins and CDKs (2). Although each member of the CKI families can inhibit CDK activity individually, they may also work cooperatively to regulate the G1/S phase progression. For instance, recent reports have suggested that CIP/KIP protein bound on CDK4 are released and re-bound to CDK2 by introducing INK4, which replaces the CIP/KIP and binds to CDK4 to cause G1 phase arrest (82-84).

Given that both classes of CDK inhibitors are essential for controlling the cell growth and DNA replication, deregulation of these molecules usually leads to malignancy. Loss of INK4 gene functions has been detected in a variety of human cancers via deletion, mutation or silencing of the chromosomal 9p21 locus (85). An INK4-CDK4/6-Rb regulatory pathway is considered essential for promoting apoptosis and senescence in cells insulted by oncogenic stimuli such as ras (86). INK4 can activate Rb and sequester E2F transcriptional factor for DNA replication, so loss of INK4 leads to Rb inactivation and carcinogenesis caused by ras over-expression. On the other hand, the CIP/KIP family members are rarely mutated or deleted in human cancers. Instead, their expressions in various cancer cells are reduced through mis-regulated post-translational stability, reduced transcription, or even microRNA (3). Although CIP/KIP family proteins are regarded as tumor suppressors because of their cell cycle regulatory role, the subcellular localizations of these proteins may alter their tumor preventive role to completely opposite functions. For example, increased cytoplasmic $p27^{KIP1}$ level has been found in tumors with higher grade, strong metastatic capacity and poor prognosis, such as breast, cervical, esophagus, uterus cancers, and leukemia/lymphoma (87-90). Also, over-expressed or mislocalized $p21^{CIP1}$ in cytoplasm is found in advanced and poor prognostic cancers including glioblastoma, carcinomas of prostate, pancreas, breast, cervix, and ovary (3, 91, 92). The underlying mechanisms are not understood, however, it has been reported that the tumor-promoting functions of CIP/KIP family proteins is likely to be associated with actin cytoskeletal organization and cancer motility (90). The RhoA signaling pathway is influenced by the cytoplasmic CIP/KIP family proteins to reorganize actin networks in cell motility. The detailed mechanisms will be described below. In addition, relocalization of CIP/KIP family proteins from the nucleus to cytoplasm may inactivate Rb by over-activated CDKs, further explain the tumor-prone manner of such a misregulation (90, 93).

Up-regulation of CIP/KIP proteins is usually detected in cells that are insulted by extracellular stimulation, such as inhibition of cell adhesion, addition or removal of mitogens, and ionizing radiation. However, the molecular mechanisms responsible for accumulation of $p21^{CIP1}$ and $p27^{KIP1}$ are not identical. Gene transactivation is the primary pathway for up-regulation of $p21^{CIP1}$. Many transcriptional responsive elements on the $p21^{CIP1}$ promoter are capable of regulating gene expression in response to different stimulations (94). For example, Sp1 sites on the $p21^{CIP1}$ gene promoter can respond to phorbol ester (PMA), histone deacetylase inhibitors (TSA), or TGF-β for gene transcription. Also, cytokines IL-6 and IFN-γ can transactivate the $p21^{CIP1}$ gene through STAT1 binding sites. In addition, ionizing radiation is able to activate wild-type p53 to transactivate the $p21^{CIP1}$ gene through the p53 consensus binding sites on the $p21^{CIP1}$ promoter (95). In response to ionizing radiation, cells with wild-type p53 up-regulates $p21^{CIP1}$ to induce G1 phase arrest (96-98). In contrast to $p21^{CIP1}$, regulation of $p27^{KIP1}$ level is dependent on posttranslational control (99). Phosphorylation of $p27^{KIP1}$ on Thr-187 is dependent on cyclin E/CDK2 and is essential for protein degradation through the ubiquitin-proteasomal mechanism (100, 101). It has been reported that SCF^{Skp2} ubiquitin ligase complex, which is composed of four major subunits (Skp1, Cul1, Rbx1/Roc1, and F-box protein Skp2), is responsible for degradation of phosphorylated $p27^{KIP1}$ (102). Inhibition of Thr-187 phosphorylation or Skp2 results in an inhibition of the entry into S phase. Also, another phosphorylation site on $p27^{KIP1}$ (Ser-10) was reported. In contrast to Thr-187, Ser-10 phosphorylation can increase the stability of $p27^{KIP1}$ protein in quiescent cells by promoting nuclear export of $p27^{KIP1}$ through CRM1/exportin1 (103-106). It can mediate the cytoplasmic relocalization of $p27^{KIP1}$ and promote cellular migration induced by hepatocyte growth factor (107). In addition to ser-10 phosphorylation, cytoplasmic localization of $p27^{KIP1}$ can be induced by phosphorylation of Thr-157 and Thr-198 mediated by Akt/PKB or p90 ribosomal S6-kinase ($p90^{RSK}$) for certain biological functions that require further investigations (89, 108, 109). Collectively, it appears that regulation of $p27^{KIP1}$ and $p21^{CIP1}$ is mediated by different pathways. Regulation of CDK activity for Rb function in different phases of cell cycle by cyclins, CKIs and other proteins is summarized in Table 1 (Table 1).

Phase	Cell cycle regulators	Molecular functions [b]	Rb activation/ inactivation
G0	INK4 (p15^{INK4a}, p16^{INK4b}, p18^{INK4c},p19^{INK4d})	Bind to and inactivate CDK4/6	activation
	p27^{kip1}	Binds to and inactivates cyclinD-CDK4 complex	activation
	cyclin C	Binds to and activates CDK3	inactivation
	cyclin D1	Binds to and activates CDK4/6	inactivation
G1	cyclin D2	Binds to and activates CDK4	inactivation
	cyclin E	Binds to and activates CDK2, can degrade p27	inactivation
	CIP/KIP (p21^{cip1}, p27^{kip1}, p57^{kip2}) [a]	Bind to and inactivate cyclin D-CDK4 or cyclin E-CDK2 complex	activation
S	cyclin A	Binds to and activates CDK2	inactivation
	cyclin D3	Binds to and activates CDK4	inactivation
G2	cyclin A	Binds to and activates CDK2	inactivation
	cyclin B1	Binds to and activates CDK1	inactivation
	p21^{cip1}	Inhibits CDK1 activity when DNA damage	activation
	Rb/histone H1 kinase	Phosphorylates the N-terminal of Rb	undetermined
Prophase	MPF	Promotes cyclin B1 synthesis	inactivation
	cyclin B1	Binds to and activates CDK1	inactivation
	MAPK	Phosphorylates Rb in Xenopus oocytes	inactivation
	cdc25	Activates CDK1 by dephosphorylation	inactivation
Metaphase	MAD2	Inhibits cyclin B1 degradation	inactivation
	BubR1	Mad2-interacting proteins for cyclin B1 degradation	activation
Anaphase	APC	Promotes cyclin B1 degradation	activation
Telophase	cdc14	Activates APC-cdh2 to promote cyclin B1 degradation	activation

a. Functions on CDK inhibition may only occur when CIP/KIP binds to cyclin/CDK with more than 1:1 stoichiometry

b. These functions are primarily included but may not be limited.

Table 1. Molecules involved in regulating CDK mediated Rb activation or inactivation

The cell cycle checkpoint is required to ensure the integrity of the genome during cell cycle progression. The function of the checkpoint is to prevent aberrant DNA from replication or chromosomal segregation. One of the most important regulators for the G1/S checkpoint is p53 (110, 111). Under normal physiological conditions, the protein level of p53 is controlled by a specific negative regulator called MDM2, which binds and promotes the degradation of the p53 protein. The activity of MDM2 can be inhibited by p19^{ARF} tumor suppressor, which is a target gene transactivated by E2F transcriptional factor (112, 113). Because release of E2F is controlled by Rb inactivation, the orchestration among the tumor suppressors and potent proto-oncogenes is important for preserving the functions of checkpoint. In response to DNA damage, p53 is phosphorylated and dissociated from MDM2. The p53 protein is subsequently resistant to degradation and accumulated in the cells (114). Accumulated p53 enters the nuclei and transactivates the downstream gene $p21^{CIP1}$ for G1 phase arrest. In the absence of p53, $p21^{CIP1}$ is not up-regulated and G1 phase arrest is abrogated after DNA damage. The molecular regulation of G1/S phase progression, including a variety of CDKs, CKIs, Rb, and p53, is illustrated in Figure 3.

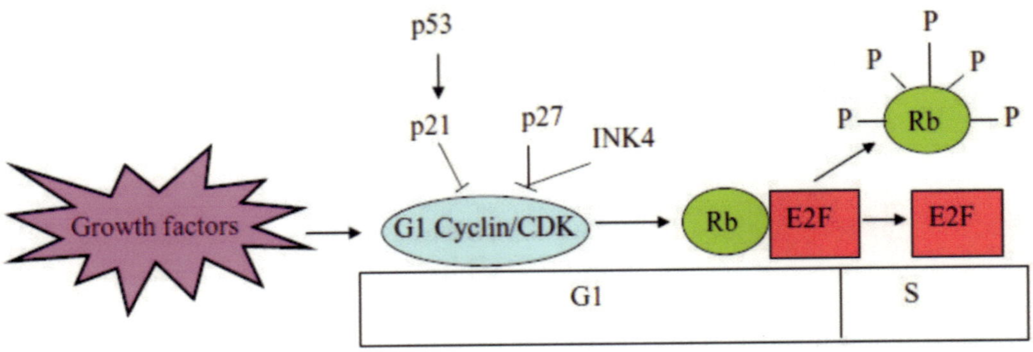

Lee YJ et al.

Fig. 3. Molecular regulation of cell cycle progression from G1 to S phase. CDK phosphorylates Rb to release E2F transcription factor for S phase entry and progression. The activity of cyclin/CDK is stimulated by growth factors and is regulated by CDK inhibitors, including $p21^{cip1}/p27^{kip1}$ and INK4 family. p53 mediates the expression of $p21^{CIP1}$ to induce G1 phase arrest, but not $p27^{KIP1}$ or INK4 family. INK4 may cooperate with $p27^{KIP1}$ to induce efficient G1 phase arrest under specific stimulation.

In adhesive cultures, cell attachment is required for entry into the cell cycle. Cells can only be stimulated by growth factor or mitogenic signals after they are anchored onto substratum. Given that actin cytoskeleton is involved in cell attachment and spreading, organization of actin structures may be important for cell cycle progression. The detailed molecular regulation through actin cytoskeletal organization and related biological events are discussed in next section.

5. Actin cytoskeleton in regulation of G1 phase progression and Rb activity

Following cytokinesis, cells enter G1 phase by the presence of growth factors that stimulate a series of signal transduction in cytosol through the surface receptors. The growth factor (or serum)-dependent cell growth includes several events: attachment onto extracellular matrix, spreading, and locomotion. These anchorage-dependent and morphology-dependent effects are important for G1 phase progression and S phase transition. Actin cytoskeletal organization is stimulated by growth factors and is involved in the mechanical and structural mediated cell cycle progression and growth (13, 115, 116). Also, the time interval of G1 phase is usually long and can be divided into early, mid, and late G1 phase in proliferating cells. The essence of actin cytoskeleton for G1 phase progression, however, is dependent on the stage of G1 phase. For instance, accumulated literatures have shown that intact actin cytoskeleton was required for mid to late G1 phase progression (116-120). Also, serum stimulation and cell anchorage may also be involved in the G1 phase progression (121). Essentially, the actin cytoskeletal organization affects Rb activity in G1 phase progression via different signaling pathways. We will elucidate the association between actin networks and Rb mediated G1 phase progression according to the literatures reviewed so far.

The organization of actin filaments is believed to be important for initiation of cell growth after cell attachment. Actin inhibitors are routinely adopted for disrupting the actin cytoskeleton in vitro and in vivo. The perturbation of cell cycle was subsequently analyzed by different approaches. The levels of G1 phase arrest were determined from DNA content measured by Feulgen or propidium iodide (PI) staining, or by 5-bromo-2′-deoxyuridine (BrdU) labeling for S phase entry after drug treatment. The significance of actin filaments is to convey the extracellular signals and form an appropriate shape for G1 phase progression (13). It is reasonable that disruption of actin filaments would lead to a G1 phase arrest. Indeed, exposure of cultured cells to sublethal concentration of actin inhibitors, such as cytochalasin or latrunculin, cause actin cytoskeletal destabilization and G1 phase arrest (117-119, 122). In some cases, cells were synchronized to G1 phase using lovastatin (118) or serum-starvation (117) before cytochalasin treatment to avoid the interference of results from cells in other phases of cell cycle. Progression of G1 cells into subsequent phases of the cell cycle was monitored after adding back mevalonate, serum or epidermal growth factor (EGF). Based on these studies, it is concluded that intact actin cytoskeleton is required for responding to extracellular stimuli after the mid-G1 phase (118). Disruption of actin cytoskeleton affects cells in passing the "restriction (R)" point for S phase entry (117, 120). Also, once cells enter S phase, the phosphorylation of Rb and CKI $p27^{KIP1}$ are not influenced by cytochalasin D treatment (118). Therefore, preservation of sufficient mechanical force for attachment and spreading by actin cytoskeleton on the solid substratum, is critical for G1 to S phase transition in anchorage-dependent cells.

The cytoskeleton formed by actin filaments is an important component for cellular adherence and cell shapes. Actin filaments are primarily concentrated beneath the plasma membrane for the formation of cortical actin cytoskeleton and actin bundles. Cell anchorage and shape formation are associated with cytoskeletal tension, and they are able to induce cyclin D1 gene transcription for inactivating Rb and promoting G1 phase progression (13, 120, 123, 124). The cyclin E/CDK2 activity in late G1 phase and S phase entry is also influenced by cell adhesion. In contrast to cyclin D1, the cyclin E and CDK2 levels do not change significantly following cell adhesion and actin cytoskeletal formation. It is likely due to reduced expression of $p21^{CIP1}$ and $p27^{KIP1}$ that can bind to and inhibit cyclinE/CDK2 complex, although other mechanisms are also involved (5, 123, 125, 126). Both cyclin D1 and cyclin E associated CDKs activity can inactivate Rb and p107 for S phase entry upon cell adhesion. Cyclin A, another important molecule responsible for S phase progression, can bind to CDK2 and replace the position occupied by cyclin E. Cell adhesion also promote cyclin A expression through E2F4-dependent or -independent mechanisms (115, 127). E2F4 is another member of E2F transcriptional factor family, and it is important for cyclin A gene transactivation (128). The E2F4-independent transactivation of cyclin A gene for S phase progression is possibly due to c-myc and CAATT binding proteins after cells attach and spread on the substratum (129, 130). Molecular regulations of cell adhesion and cell shape changes in G1 phase progression can be blocked by actin inhibitors that induce destabilization of actin cytoskeleton. The effects of actin cytoskeletal destabilization on cell cycle progression are usually consistent with the results of cells cultured in suspension or cell spreading is limited by microfabricated substrates containing fibronectin-coated adhesive islands (116, 121, 124).

Intact actin cytoskeleton is important for Rb inactivation by releasing the E2F transcriptional factor for promoting DNA replication. However, the pathways that mediate actin inhibitors induced actin cytoskeletal destabilization are diverse. For instance, Huang and Ingber proposed that cytochalasin D causes down-regulation of cyclin D1 and up-regulation of $p27^{KIP1}$ (118). Reshetnikova et al. found that dihydrocytochalasin B inhibited the expression of cyclin E but not cyclin D1 in Swiss 3T3 cells (117). However, the levels of $p21^{CIP1}$ and $p27^{KIP1}$ were not affected under the same treatment. Fasshauer et al. suggested that disorganization of actin filaments using latrunculin A, latrunculin B, or cytochalasin D leads to reduction of c-jun and cyclin (D1, E, A) expression and inhibition of entry into S phase (131). Interestingly, Rb and p107 double-null mouse embryo fibroblasts (MEFs) are able to reach mid-G1 phase without serum stimulation, whereas they can not transit to the S phase without anchorage (121). This observation is based on a comparison of the expression of cyclin E in Rb-/-p107-/- cells between normal attachment and suspension cultured conditions. Growth factor stimulation, cytoskeletal organization and cell anchorage are essential for cyclin D1 induction and Rb phosphorylation until mid-G1 phase (121, 132, 133). Disruption of actin cytoskeleton leads to dephosphorylation and activation of Rb in wild-type cells but not in RB pocket proteins-null cells. In agreement, a TKO MEF with deletions of all Rb pocket proteins exhibits impaired G1 phase arrest and aneuploidy following disruption of actin cytoskeleton (134). In addition, Rho small GTPase protein mediated signaling pathway is involved in actin stress fiber formation, $p27^{KIP1}$ degradation and cyclin D1 expression, which promotes Rb inactivation as well as cyclin E/CDK2 activation for entry of the G1 phase (132, 133, 135). Together, although the molecular events for actin cytoskeletal regulated G1 phase progression may be different among cell types, Rb family protein can be regarded as a common checkpoint molecule that allows cells with intact actin cytoskeleton passing through the G1 to S phase (Figure 4).

Several lines of evidence have shown that actin cytoskeleton may be important for cytoplasmic localization of tumor suppressor p53 during the cell cycle progression (136-138). Sequestration of p53 in the cytoplasmic portion is important for prevention of cell cycle arrest and apoptosis under normal cell growth (139). Activation of p53 by cytochalasin D was also reported, while this effect is associated with drug induced apoptosis (140). In addition, cytochalasin B can induce DNA fragmentation in specific cell types (141). On the other hand, disruption of actin cytoskeleton induced G1 phase arrest has been reported to be associated with Rb pocket protein rather than p53 activation (134). We also demonstrated that actin inhibitors induced a p53-independent up-regulation of $p21^{CIP1}$ in various mammalian p53-null cancer cell lines (142). Up-regulated $p21^{CIP1}$ is dependent on a post-translational pathway to increase the protein stability and activate Rb for the G1 phase arrest. The response of $p27^{KIP1}$ is relatively weak under the same condition of treatment. Taken together, it appears that different drugs used for disruption of actin filaments can activate different pathways to cause G1 phase arrest. Induction of p53-independent G1 phase arrest by actin inhibitors is especially interesting because p53 tumor suppressor is frequently inactivated or mutated in human cancers. The Rb tumor suppressor may play an important role in mediating the actin cytoskeletal destabilization that causes G1 phase arrest. It is also of interest to further investigate the crosstalk between $p21^{CIP1}$ and Rb regarding toxins-induced actin cytoskeletal destabilization.

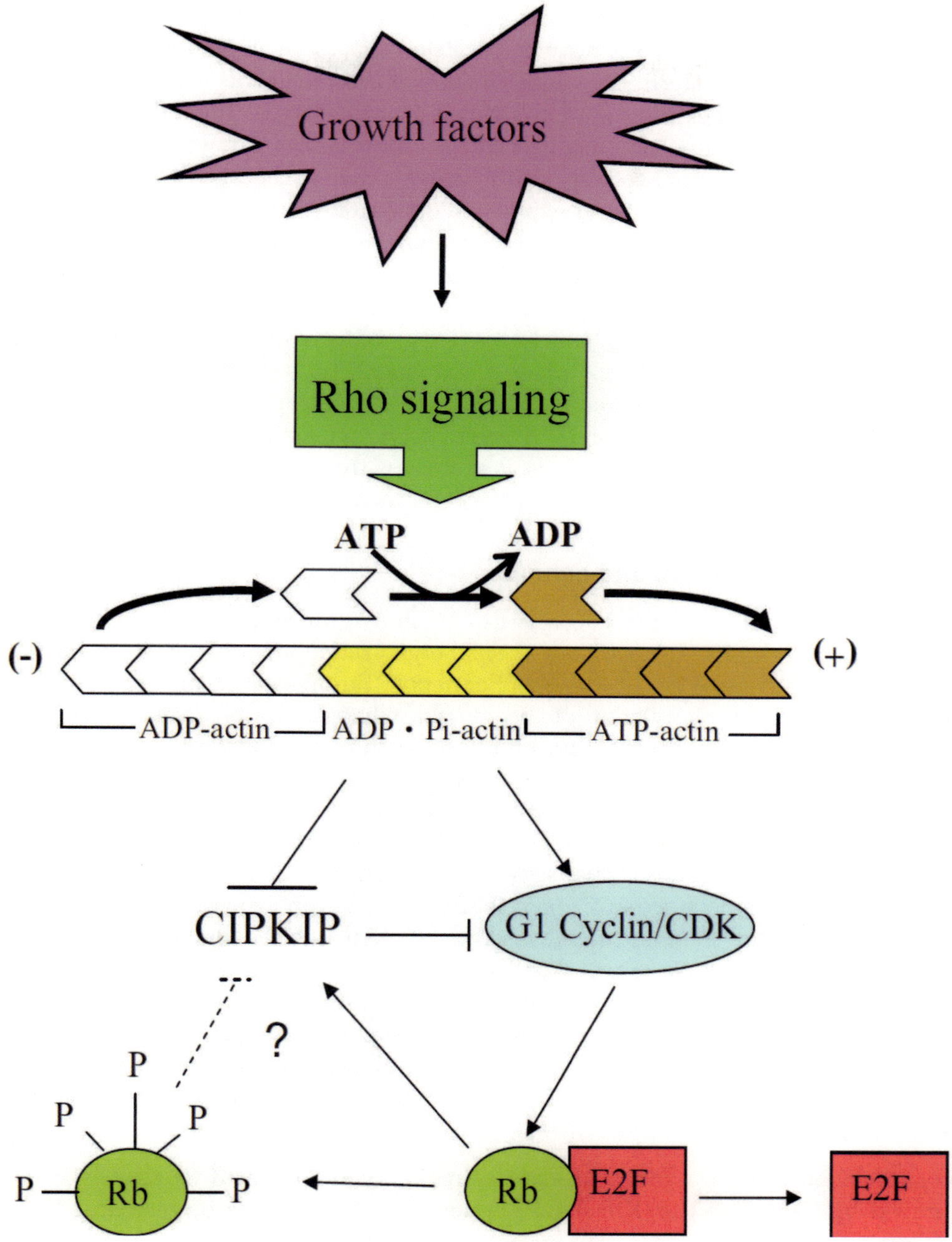

Lee YJ et al.

Fig. 4. Growth factor stimulated Rb inactivation is mediated by the actin cytoskeletal integrity. Intact actin cytoskeleton organized by the Rho signaling pathway leads to a repression of CIP/KIP family proteins and increase of G1 phase associated cyclin/CDKs activity, which can inactivate Rb by serine/threonine phosphorylation (P). Activated Rb may increase $p27^{KIP1}$ stability through a down-regulation of Skp2 gene (see text). Whether inactivated Rb can oppositely inhibit CIP/KIP proteins remains an opening question.

To avoid unexpected side-effects raised by actin toxins, use of actin regulatory proteins for molecular-based destabilization of actin cytoskeleton should be an interesting approach to investigate the cell cycle effect. Since the formation of actin filaments is regulated by actin-binding proteins, forced expression of the related proteins may be able to destabilize actin filaments and influence the cell cycle distribution. Indeed, over-expression of gelsolin, an actin-regulatory protein, has been reported to activate the G2 checkpoint in human cancer cells by gene transfection (143). Over-expression of G-actin sequestrating protein thymosin β–4 also caused S and G2/M phase arrest in human colon cancers (144). Moreover, over-expression of profilin-1, an actin polymerizing molecule, induces G1 phase arrest in MDA-MB-231 breast cancer cell line through $p27^{KIP1}$ stabilization (145). In our lab, we focused on actin dynamic regulator cofilin-1 and showed that induction of cofilin-1 expression in human lung cancer cells led to a G1 phase arrest via $p27^{KIP1}$ regulatory pathways (39, 40). Also, Rb phosphorylation is apparently reduced by forced expression of cofilin-1. Although destabilization of actin cytoskeleton by different actin regulatory proteins may inhibit cell cycle progression through distinct routes, it is obvious that actin cytoskeleton is important for cancer cells and would be an important target for therapeutic design.

6. Rb, actin cytoskeleton, and cancer

Rb is a tumor suppressor gene, which is usually loss-of-function in a broad spectrum of human cancers (146, 147). The actin cytoskeletal organization induced cyclin D1 expression and CDK activity is essential for Rb phosphorylation. Destabilization of actin cytoskeleton activates Rb by dephosphorylation of the protein, whereas loss of Rb may abrogate G1 phase arrest and lead to aneuploidy for rapid cell death (134). Therefore, it seems plausible that actin inhibitors are ideal for the treatment of Rb-deficient cancers. Several different classes of actin inhibitors, such as cytochalasin and latrunculin, have been subjected to the clinical chemotherapy trial (148, 149). Because Rb is not mutated in normal tissues, these actin inhibitors may exhibit selective activities between the cancer mass and surrounding tissues. Moreover, we have recently found that latrunculin can increase the radiosensitivity in human lung cancer cell lines (unpublished data). Although the underlying mechanisms remain to be addressed, we expect that latrunculin can be used as a radiosensitizer for cancer treatment. In fact, we have shown that over-expression of cofilin-1 can destabilize actin architectures and increase the cellular radiosensitivity by suppressing the DNA repair capacity (150). Up-regulation of cofilin-1 was also found in cells exposed to latrunculin (unpublished data), suggesting that actin inhibitor can suppress cytoskeletal dynamics and DNA damage responses consequently.

Phosphorylation of Rb is mainly dependent on G1 cyclin associated CDKs, which is also controlled by CKIs. The CIP/KIP family proteins are found to be up-regulated by actin inhibitors. The stabilities rather than mRNA levels of these proteins are usually increased after destabilization of actin cytoskeleton or by limiting the cell anchorage and spreading. It has been reported that $p27^{KIP1}$ coordinates with CDK and Rb to control the proliferation and migration in vascular smooth muscle cells and fibroblasts (151). Interestingly, recent studies propose that Rb can reversely influence the $p27^{KIP1}$ expression through inhibition of Skp2, a pivotal molecule required for $p27^{KIP1}$ degradation (4, 152). Analysis of the promoter of Skp2 gene showed that an E2F binding site was essential for gene transcription (4). Therefore, it becomes clear that $p27^{KIP1}$ level should be ablated by Rb-E2F during G1/S phase transition depending on the cyclin E/CDK2 activity. Activation of Rb is sufficient to suppress Skp2 expression and increase $p27^{KIP1}$ stability. Therefore, it is speculated that disruption of actin cytoskeleton can also trigger the Rb-Skp2-$p27^{KIP1}$ auto-regulatory circuit and inhibit G1/S phase transition. Skp2 has been found to be over-expressed in several cancers (153, 154). Targeting on Skp2 has been reported to suppress the tumorigenesis (155). Whether use of actin inhibitors can also repress Skp2 expression would be an interesting direction for investigation. In Rb-deficiency cancer cells, disruption of actin cytoskeleton may overlook the checkpoint by excessive suppression of $p27^{KIP1}$ expression for apoptosis (134). Over-expressed Skp2, although it may promote tumorigenesis, may become a reversed knife to induce death of cancer lacking Rb expression following disruption of actin architectures.

Metastasis is the primary cause of cancer mortality, and Rho-mediated actin reorganization is believed to be essential for enhanced cancer cell motility. The CIP/KIP family proteins have been reported to regulate molecules of Rho signaling pathway when they are relocalized to the cytoplasm from the nucleus (3). For instance, $p27^{KIP1}$ can bind to Rho small GTPase (93), $p21^{CIP1}$ binds to Rho kinase (ROCK) (156) and $p57^{kip2}$ binds to LIMK for actin reorganization (157). All of these events may increase cell motility by activating cofilin-1 for promoting the actin dynamics at the leading edges. Also, lack of nuclear CIP/KIP proteins may concomitantly inactivate Rb and enhance cell cycle progression. Whether disruption of actin cytoskeleton can affect cytoplasmic CIP/KIP and subsequently reactivate Rb is of interest to be further investigated. It is speculated that reactivation of Rb by nuclear relocalization of CIP/KIP proteins in cancer cells can be achieved by treatment with actin inhibitors.

7. Conclusion and perspectives

More than five thousand of research publications have been dedicated to Rb and tumorigenesis in the passed two decades. As the first identified tumor suppressor gene, it is no doubt that Rb is an important target for designing new cancer therapeutic agents. Studies of actin cytoskeletal organization in cell anchorage and spreading have greatly improved the understanding of the relationship between growth factors mediated cell cycle progression and Rb inactivation. Since disruption of actin cytoskeleton is known to activate Rb and block G1 phase progression, the actin inhibitors may prevent cancer growth. Especially, activated Rb can repress Skp2 oncogene and increase the stability of $p27^{KIP1}$, which is a consequence of actin cytoskeletal disruption. Also, actin inhibitors may promote aneuploidy and death in Rb-deficient cancer cells. Although targeting on actin cytoskeleton and consequent Rb-related pathways provides a promising future in cancer treatment, several critical problems remain to be noticed and addressed: (1) It is not clear whether actin inhibitors can efficiently distinguish the malignancy from normal tissues? What is the optimal dose for cancer prevention with minimum damage to normal tissues? (2) Will actin inhibitors induce genomic instability and mutation in malignancy, especially for those that lack Rb expression? (3) Since actin inhibitors not only block G1 phase progression but also G2/M and cytokinesis, it is unclear whether Rb is also involved in the checkpoints of different phases of the cell cycle after actin inhibitor treatment? (4) It is of interest to know whether actin inhibitors can affect the expression or activity of actin-binding proteins on the cell cycle perturbation. Do actin inhibitors affect Rb activity through signaling pathways that regulates specific actin-binding proteins? (5) Does altered expression of actin-binding proteins influence Rb activity? If yes, what are the potential molecular mechanisms? These questions are involved but not limited to the further exploration of the interactions between actin cytoskeletal organization and Rb biology. It is believed that a comprehensive study of actin skeleton and Rb, and related pathways and mechanisms will broaden the view of Rb biology on cancer treatment.

8. Acknowledgments

This chapter was granted by National Science Council of Taiwan, R.O.C. (NSC99-2314-B-010-029-MY3)

9. References

[1] Frixione E: Recurring views on the structure and function of the cytoskeleton: a 300-year epic. Cell Motil Cytoskeleton. *46(2)*: 73-94, 2000.
[2] Sherr CJ and Roberts JM: CDK inhibitors: positive and negative regulators of G1-phase progression. Genes Dev. *13(12)*: 1501-1512, 1999.
[3] Besson A, Dowdy SF and Roberts JM: CDK inhibitors: cell cycle regulators and beyond. Dev Cell. *14(2)*: 159-169, 2008.
[4] Yung Y, Walker JL, Roberts JM and Assoian RK: A Skp2 autoinduction loop and restriction point control. J Cell Biol. *178(5)*: 741-747, 2007.
[5] Fang F, Orend G, Watanabe N, Hunter T and Ruoslahti E: Dependence of cyclin E-CDK2 kinase activity on cell anchorage. Science. *271(5248)*: 499-502, 1996.
[6] Tapon N and Hall A: Rho, Rac and Cdc42 GTPases regulate the organization of the actin cytoskeleton. Curr Opin Cell Biol. *9(1)*: 86-92, 1997.
[7] Burridge K, Fath K, Kelly T, Nuckolls G and Turner C: Focal adhesions: transmembrane junctions between the extracellular matrix and the cytoskeleton. Annu Rev Cell Biol. *4(*487-525, 1988.
[8] Schlaepfer DD and Hunter T: Signal transduction from the extracellular matrix--a role for the focal adhesion protein-tyrosine kinase FAK. Cell Struct Funct. *21(5)*: 445-450, 1996.
[9] Chen HC, Appeddu PA, Isoda H and Guan JL: Phosphorylation of tyrosine 397 in focal adhesion kinase is required for binding phosphatidylinositol 3-kinase. J Biol Chem. *271(42)*: 26329-26334, 1996.
[10] Zhao JH, Reiske H and Guan JL: Regulation of the cell cycle by focal adhesion kinase. J Cell Biol. *143(7)*: 1997-2008, 1998.
[11] Chen Q, Kinch MS, Lin TH, Burridge K and Juliano RL: Integrin-mediated cell adhesion activates mitogen-activated protein kinases. J Biol Chem. *269(43)*: 26602-26605, 1994.
[12] Yamada KM and Miyamoto S: Integrin transmembrane signaling and cytoskeletal control. Curr Opin Cell Biol. *7(5)*: 681-689, 1995.
[13] Assoian RK and Zhu X: Cell anchorage and the cytoskeleton as partners in growth factor dependent cell cycle progression. Curr Opin Cell Biol. *9(1)*: 93-98, 1997.
[14] Maness PF and Walsh RC, Jr.: Dihydrocytochalasin B disorganizes actin cytoarchitecture and inhibits initiation of DNA synthesis in 3T3 cells. Cell. *30(1)*: 253-262, 1982.
[15] Strome S: Determination of cleavage planes. Cell. *72(1)*: 3-6, 1993.

[16] Guizetti J and Gerlich DW: Cytokinetic abscission in animal cells. Semin Cell Dev Biol. *21(9)*: 909-916, 2010.

[17] Kondo T, Hamao K, Kamijo K, Kimura H, Morita M, Takahashi M and Hosoya H: Enhancement of myosin II/actin turnover at the contractile ring induces slower furrowing in dividing HeLa cells. Biochem J. *435(3)*: 569-576, 2011.

[18] Robinson DN and Spudich JA: Mechanics and regulation of cytokinesis. Curr Opin Cell Biol. *16(2)*: 182-188, 2004.

[19] Clayton L and Lloyd CW: Actin organization during the cell cycle in meristematic plant cells. Actin is present in the cytokinetic phragmoplast. Exp Cell Res. *156(1)*: 231-238, 1985.

[20] Seagull RW, Falconer MM and Weerdenburg CA: Microfilaments: dynamic arrays in higher plant cells. J Cell Biol. *104(4)*: 995-1004, 1987.

[21] Tiwari SC, Wick SM, Williamson RE and Gunning BE: Cytoskeleton and integration of cellular function in cells of higher plants. J Cell Biol. *99(1 Pt 2)*: 63s-69s, 1984.

[22] Palevitz BA: Actin in the preprophase band of Allium cepa. J Cell Biol. *104(6)*: 1515-1519, 1987.

[23] Sanger JW and Holtzer H: Cytochalasin-B: effects on cytokinesis, glycogen and 3 H-D-gluconse incorporation. Am J Anat. *135(2)*: 293-298, 1972.

[24] Estensen RD: Cytochalasin B. I. Effect on cytokinesis of Novikoff hepatoma cells. Proc Soc Exp Biol Med. *136(4)*: 1256-1260, 1971.

[25] Estensen RD, Rosenberg M, Sheridan JD, Wessells NK, Spooner BS, Ash JF, Luduena MA and Wrenn JT: Cytochalasin B: microfilaments and "contractile" processes. Science. *173(3994)*: 356-359, 1971.

[26] Ji JY, Haghnia M, Trusty C, Goldstein LS and Schubiger G: A genetic screen for suppressors and enhancers of the Drosophila cdk1-cyclin B identifies maternal factors that regulate microtubule and microfilament stability. Genetics. *162(3)*: 1179-1195, 2002.

[27] von Dassow G and Schubiger G: How an actin network might cause fountain streaming and nuclear migration in the syncytial Drosophila embryo. J Cell Biol. *127(6 Pt 1)*: 1637-1653, 1994.

[28] Cowan CR and Hyman AA: Acto-myosin reorganization and PAR polarity in C. elegans. Development. *134(6)*: 1035-1043, 2007.

[29] Na J and Zernicka-Goetz M: Asymmetric positioning and organization of the meiotic spindle of mouse oocytes requires CDC42 function. Curr Biol. *16(12)*: 1249-1254, 2006.

[30] Schuh M and Ellenberg J: A new model for asymmetric spindle positioning in mouse oocytes. Curr Biol. *18(24)*: 1986-1992, 2008.

[31] Wang L, Wang ZB, Zhang X, FitzHarris G, Baltz JM, Sun QY and Liu XJ: Brefeldin A disrupts asymmetric spindle positioning in mouse oocytes. Dev Biol. *313(1)*: 155-166, 2008.

[32] Woolner S, O'Brien LL, Wiese C and Bement WM: Myosin-10 and actin filaments are essential for mitotic spindle function. J Cell Biol. *182(1)*: 77-88, 2008.

[33] Lenart P, Bacher CP, Daigle N, Hand AR, Eils R, Terasaki M and Ellenberg J: A contractile nuclear actin network drives chromosome congression in oocytes. Nature. *436(7052)*: 812-818, 2005.

[34] Kunda P and Baum B: The actin cytoskeleton in spindle assembly and positioning. Trends Cell Biol. *19(4)*: 174-179, 2009.

[35] Gachet Y, Tournier S, Millar JB and Hyams JS: A MAP kinase-dependent actin checkpoint ensures proper spindle orientation in fission yeast. Nature. *412(6844)*: 352-355, 2001.

[36] Schmit AC and Lambert AM: Characterization and dynamics of cytoplasmic F-actin in higher plant endosperm cells during interphase, mitosis, and cytokinesis. J Cell Biol. *105(5)*: 2157-2166, 1987.

[37] Gurniak CB, Perlas E and Witke W: The actin depolymerizing factor n-cofilin is essential for neural tube morphogenesis and neural crest cell migration. Dev Biol. *278(1)*: 231-241, 2005.

[38] Bellenchi GC, Gurniak CB, Perlas E, Middei S, Ammassari-Teule M and Witke W: N-cofilin is associated with neuronal migration disorders and cell cycle control in the cerebral cortex. Genes Dev. *21(18)*: 2347-2357, 2007.

[39] Tsai CH, Chiu SJ, Liu CC, Sheu TJ, Hsieh CH, Keng PC and Lee YJ: Regulated expression of cofilin and the consequent regulation of p27(kip1) are essential for G(1) phase progression. Cell Cycle. *8(15)*: 2365-2374, 2009.

[40] Lee YJ and Keng PC: Studying the effects of actin cytoskeletal destabilization on cell cycle by cofilin overexpression. Mol Biotechnol. *31(1)*: 1-10, 2005.

[41] Peter M, Heitlinger E, Haner M, Aebi U and Nigg EA: Disassembly of in vitro formed lamin head-to-tail polymers by CDC2 kinase. Embo J. *10(6)*: 1535-1544, 1991.

[42] Hartwell LH and Kastan MB: Cell cycle control and cancer. Science. *266(5192)*: 1821-1828, 1994.

[43] Cheng M, Olivier P, Diehl JA, Fero M, Roussel MF, Roberts JM and Sherr CJ: The p21(Cip1) and p27(Kip1) CDK 'inhibitors' are essential activators of cyclin D-dependent kinases in murine fibroblasts. EMBO J. *18(6)*: 1571-1583, 1999.

[44] Ren S and Rollins BJ: Cyclin C/cdk3 promotes Rb-dependent G0 exit. Cell. *117(2)*: 239-251, 2004.

[45] Bartek J and Lukas J: Are all cancer genes equal? Nature. *411(6841)*: 1001-1002, 2001.

[46] Gjetting T, Lukas J, Bartek J and Strauss M: Regulated expression of the retinoblastoma susceptibility gene in mammary carcinoma cells restores cyclin D1 expression and G1-phase control. Biol Chem Hoppe Seyler. *376(7)*: 441-446, 1995.

[47] Lukas J, Bartkova J, Rohde M, Strauss M and Bartek J: Cyclin D1 is dispensable for G1 control in retinoblastoma gene-deficient cells independently of cdk4 activity. Mol Cell Biol. *15(5)*: 2600-2611, 1995.

[48] Nevins JR: The Rb/E2F pathway and cancer. Hum Mol Genet. *10(7)*: 699-703, 2001.

[49] Lundberg AS and Weinberg RA: Functional inactivation of the retinoblastoma protein requires sequential modification by at least two distinct cyclin-cdk complexes. Mol Cell Biol. *18(2)*: 753-761, 1998.

[50] DeGregori J, Kowalik T and Nevins JR: Cellular targets for activation by the E2F1 transcription factor include DNA synthesis- and G1/S-regulatory genes. Mol Cell Biol. *15(8)*: 4215-4224, 1995.

[51] Stanelle J, Stiewe T, Theseling CC, Peter M and Putzer BM: Gene expression changes in response to E2F1 activation. Nucleic Acids Res. *30(8)*: 1859-1867, 2002.

[52] Knudsen ES and Wang JY: Dual mechanisms for the inhibition of E2F binding to RB by cyclin-dependent kinase-mediated RB phosphorylation. Mol Cell Biol. *17(10)*: 5771-5783, 1997.

[53] Chew YP, Ellis M, Wilkie S and Mittnacht S: pRB phosphorylation mutants reveal role of pRB in regulating S phase completion by a mechanism independent of E2F. Oncogene. *17(17)*: 2177-2186, 1998.

[54] Sever-Chroneos Z, Angus SP, Fribourg AF, Wan H, Todorov I, Knudsen KE and Knudsen ES: Retinoblastoma tumor suppressor protein signals through inhibition of cyclin-dependent kinase 2 activity to disrupt PCNA function in S phase. Mol Cell Biol. *21(12)*: 4032-4045, 2001.

[55] Masselli A and Wang JY: Phosphorylation site mutated RB exerts contrasting effects on apoptotic response to different stimuli. Oncogene. *25(9)*: 1290-1298, 2006.

[56] Wang JY, Naderi S and Chen TT: Role of retinoblastoma tumor suppressor protein in DNA damage response. Acta Oncol. *40(6)*: 689-695, 2001.

[57] Wang S, Nath N, Minden A and Chellappan S: Regulation of Rb and E2F by signal transduction cascades: divergent effects of JNK1 and p38 kinases. EMBO J. *18(6)*: 1559-1570, 1999.

[58] Dasgupta P, Sun J, Wang S, Fusaro G, Betts V, Padmanabhan J, Sebti SM and Chellappan SP: Disruption of the Rb--Raf-1 interaction inhibits tumor growth and angiogenesis. Mol Cell Biol. *24(21)*: 9527-9541, 2004.

[59] Nath N, Wang S, Betts V, Knudsen E and Chellappan S: Apoptotic and mitogenic stimuli inactivate Rb by differential utilization of p38 and cyclin-dependent kinases. Oncogene. *22(38)*: 5986-5994, 2003.

[60] Singh S, Johnson J and Chellappan S: Small molecule regulators of Rb-E2F pathway as modulators of transcription. Biochim Biophys Acta. *1799(10-12)*: 788-794, 2010.

[61] Naderi S, Hunton IC and Wang JY: Radiation dose-dependent maintenance of G(2) arrest requires retinoblastoma protein. Cell Cycle. *1(3)*: 193-200, 2002.

[62] Santamaria D, Barriere C, Cerqueira A, Hunt S, Tardy C, Newton K, Caceres JF, Dubus P, Malumbres M and Barbacid M: Cdk1 is sufficient to drive the mammalian cell cycle. Nature. *448(7155)*: 811-815, 2007.

[63] Ludlow JW, Glendening CL, Livingston DM and DeCarprio JA: Specific enzymatic dephosphorylation of the retinoblastoma protein. Mol Cell Biol. *13(1)*: 367-372, 1993.

[64] Sterner JM, Murata Y, Kim HG, Kennett SB, Templeton DJ and Horowitz JM: Detection of a novel cell cycle-regulated kinase activity that associates with the amino terminus of the retinoblastoma protein in G2/M phases. J Biol Chem. *270(16)*: 9281-9288, 1995.

[65] Sterner JM, Tao Y, Kennett SB, Kim HG and Horowitz JM: The amino terminus of the retinoblastoma (Rb) protein associates with a cyclin-dependent kinase-like kinase via Rb amino acids required for growth suppression. Cell Growth Differ. *7(1)*: 53-64, 1996.

[66] Cobrinik D: Pocket proteins and cell cycle control. Oncogene. *24(17)*: 2796-2809, 2005.

[67] Sherr CJ and McCormick F: The RB and p53 pathways in cancer. Cancer Cell. *2(2)*: 103-112, 2002.

[68] Saddic LA, West LE, Aslanian A, Yates JR, 3rd, Rubin SM, Gozani O and Sage J: Methylation of the retinoblastoma tumor suppressor by SMYD2. J Biol Chem. *285(48)*: 37733-37740, 2010.

[69] Ianari A and Gulino A: Cell death or survival: the complex choice of the retinoblastoma tumor suppressor protein. Cell Cycle. *9(1)*: 23-24, 2010.

[70] Sharma A, Yeow WS, Ertel A, Coleman I, Clegg N, Thangavel C, Morrissey C, Zhang X, Comstock CE, Witkiewicz AK, Gomella L, Knudsen ES, Nelson PS and Knudsen KE: The retinoblastoma tumor suppressor controls androgen signaling and human prostate cancer progression. J Clin Invest. *120(12)*: 4478-4492, 2010.

[71] Knudsen ES and Knudsen KE: Retinoblastoma tumor suppressor: where cancer meets the cell cycle. Exp Biol Med (Maywood). *231(7)*: 1271-1281, 2006.

[72] Knudsen ES, Sexton CR and Mayhew CN: Role of the retinoblastoma tumor suppressor in the maintenance of genome integrity. Curr Mol Med. *6(7)*: 749-757, 2006.

[73] Lee JO, Russo AA and Pavletich NP: Structure of the retinoblastoma tumour-suppressor pocket domain bound to a peptide from HPV E7. Nature. *391(6670)*: 859-865, 1998.

[74] Dunaief JL, Strober BE, Guha S, Khavari PA, Alin K, Luban J, Begemann M, Crabtree GR and Goff SP: The retinoblastoma protein and BRG1 form a complex and cooperate to induce cell cycle arrest. Cell. *79(1)*: 119-130, 1994.

[75] Singh P, Coe J and Hong W: A role for retinoblastoma protein in potentiating transcriptional activation by the glucocorticoid receptor. Nature. *374(6522)*: 562-565, 1995.

[76] Gray SG, Iglesias AH, Lizcano F, Villanueva R, Camelo S, Jingu H, Teh BT, Koibuchi N, Chin WW, Kokkotou E and Dangond F: Functional characterization of JMJD2A, a histone deacetylase- and retinoblastoma-binding protein. J Biol Chem. *280(31)*: 28507-28518, 2005.

[77] Chen D, Pacal M, Wenzel P, Knoepfler PS, Leone G and Bremner R: Division and apoptosis of E2f-deficient retinal progenitors. Nature. *462(7275)*: 925-929, 2009.

[78] Zhang H, Xiong Y and Beach D: Proliferating cell nuclear antigen and p21 are components of multiple cell cycle kinase complexes. Mol Biol Cell. *4(9)*: 897-906, 1993.

[79] Polyak K, Lee MH, Erdjument-Bromage H, Koff A, Roberts JM, Tempst P and Massague J: Cloning of p27Kip1, a cyclin-dependent kinase inhibitor and a potential mediator of extracellular antimitogenic signals. Cell. *78(1)*: 59-66, 1994.

[80] Toyoshima H and Hunter T: p27, a novel inhibitor of G1 cyclin-Cdk protein kinase activity, is related to p21. Cell. *78(1)*: 67-74, 1994.

[81] Xiong Y, Zhang H and Beach D: Subunit rearrangement of the cyclin-dependent kinases is associated with cellular transformation. Genes Dev. *7(8)*: 1572-1583, 1993.

[82] Parry DA and Steinert PM: Intermediate filaments: molecular architecture, assembly, dynamics and polymorphism. Q Rev Biophys. *32(2)*: 99-187, 1999.

[83] Reynisdottir I and Massague J: The subcellular locations of p15(Ink4b) and p27(Kip1) coordinate their inhibitory interactions with cdk4 and cdk2. Genes Dev. *11(4)*: 492-503, 1997.

[84] McConnell BB, Gregory FJ, Stott FJ, Hara E and Peters G: Induced expression of p16(INK4a) inhibits both CDK4- and CDK2-associated kinase activity by reassortment of cyclin-CDK-inhibitor complexes. Mol Cell Biol. *19(3)*: 1981-1989, 1999.

[85] Canepa ET, Scassa ME, Ceruti JM, Marazita MC, Carcagno AL, Sirkin PF and Ogara MF: INK4 proteins, a family of mammalian CDK inhibitors with novel biological functions. IUBMB Life. *59(7)*: 419-426, 2007.

[86] Zou X, Ray D, Aziyu A, Christov K, Boiko AD, Gudkov AV and Kiyokawa H: Cdk4 disruption renders primary mouse cells resistant to oncogenic transformation, leading to Arf/p53-independent senescence. Genes Dev. *16(22)*: 2923-2934, 2002.

[87] Slingerland J and Pagano M: Regulation of the cdk inhibitor p27 and its deregulation in cancer. J Cell Physiol. *183(1)*: 10-17, 2000.

[88] Philipp-Staheli J, Payne SR and Kemp CJ: p27(Kip1): regulation and function of a haploinsufficient tumor suppressor and its misregulation in cancer. Exp Cell Res. *264(1)*: 148-168, 2001.

[89] Liang J, Zubovitz J, Petrocelli T, Kotchetkov R, Connor MK, Han K, Lee JH, Ciarallo S, Catzavelos C, Beniston R, Franssen E and Slingerland JM: PKB/Akt phosphorylates p27, impairs nuclear import of p27 and opposes p27-mediated G1 arrest. Nat Med. *8(10)*: 1153-1160, 2002.

[90] Besson A, Assoian RK and Roberts JM: Regulation of the cytoskeleton: an oncogenic function for CDK inhibitors? Nat Rev Cancer. *4(12)*: 948-955, 2004.

[91] Biankin AV, Kench JG, Morey AL, Lee CS, Biankin SA, Head DR, Hugh TB, Henshall SM and Sutherland RL: Overexpression of p21(WAF1/CIP1) is an early event in the development of pancreatic intraepithelial neoplasia. Cancer Res. *61(24)*: 8830-8837, 2001.

[92] Roninson IB: Oncogenic functions of tumour suppressor p21(Waf1/Cip1/Sdi1): association with cell senescence and tumour-promoting activities of stromal fibroblasts. Cancer Lett. *179(1)*: 1-14, 2002.

[93] Besson A, Gurian-West M, Schmidt A, Hall A and Roberts JM: p27Kip1 modulates cell migration through the regulation of RhoA activation. Genes Dev. *18(8)*: 862-876, 2004.

[94] Gartel AL and Tyner AL: Transcriptional regulation of the p21((WAF1/CIP1)) gene. Exp Cell Res. *246(2)*: 280-289, 1999.

[95] el-Deiry WS, Tokino T, Velculescu VE, Levy DB, Parsons R, Trent JM, Lin D, Mercer WE, Kinzler KW and Vogelstein B: WAF1, a potential mediator of p53 tumor suppression. Cell. *75(4)*: 817-825, 1993.

[96] Macleod KF, Sherry N, Hannon G, Beach D, Tokino T, Kinzler K, Vogelstein B and Jacks T: p53-dependent and independent expression of p21 during cell growth, differentiation, and DNA damage. Genes Dev. *9(8)*: 935-944, 1995.

[97] Namba H, Hara T, Tukazaki T, Migita K, Ishikawa N, Ito K, Nagataki S and Yamashita S: Radiation-induced G1 arrest is selectively mediated by the p53-WAF1/Cip1 pathway in human thyroid cells. Cancer Res. *55(10)*: 2075-2080, 1995.

[98] Dulic V, Kaufmann WK, Wilson SJ, Tlsty TD, Lees E, Harper JW, Elledge SJ and Reed SI: p53-dependent inhibition of cyclin-dependent kinase activities in human fibroblasts during radiation-induced G1 arrest. Cell. *76(6)*: 1013-1023, 1994.

[99] Nakayama K: Cip/Kip cyclin-dependent kinase inhibitors: brakes of the cell cycle engine during development. Bioessays. *20(12)*: 1020-1029, 1998.

[100] Sheaff RJ, Groudine M, Gordon M, Roberts JM and Clurman BE: Cyclin E-CDK2 is a regulator of p27Kip1. Genes Dev. *11(11)*: 1464-1478, 1997.

[101] Pagano M, Tam SW, Theodoras AM, Beer-Romero P, Del Sal G, Chau V, Yew PR, Draetta GF and Rolfe M: Role of the ubiquitin-proteasome pathway in regulating abundance of the cyclin-dependent kinase inhibitor p27. Science. *269(5224)*: 682-685, 1995.

[102] Carrano AC and Pagano M: Role of the F-box protein Skp2 in adhesion-dependent cell cycle progression. J Cell Biol. *153(7)*: 1381-1390, 2001.

[103] Ishida N, Kitagawa M, Hatakeyama S and Nakayama K: Phosphorylation at serine 10, a major phosphorylation site of p27(Kip1), increases its protein stability. J Biol Chem. *275(33)*: 25146-25154, 2000.

[104] Besson A, Gurian-West M, Chen X, Kelly-Spratt KS, Kemp CJ and Roberts JM: A pathway in quiescent cells that controls p27Kip1 stability, subcellular localization, and tumor suppression. Genes Dev. *20(1)*: 47-64, 2006.

[105] Connor MK, Kotchetkov R, Cariou S, Resch A, Lupetti R, Beniston RG, Melchior F, Hengst L and Slingerland JM: CRM1/Ran-mediated nuclear export of p27(Kip1)

involves a nuclear export signal and links p27 export and proteolysis. Mol Biol Cell. *14(1)*: 201-213, 2003.

[106] Rodier G, Montagnoli A, Di Marcotullio L, Coulombe P, Draetta GF, Pagano M and Meloche S: p27 cytoplasmic localization is regulated by phosphorylation on Ser10 and is not a prerequisite for its proteolysis. EMBO J. *20(23)*: 6672-6682, 2001.

[107] McAllister SS, Becker-Hapak M, Pintucci G, Pagano M and Dowdy SF: Novel p27(kip1) C-terminal scatter domain mediates Rac-dependent cell migration independent of cell cycle arrest functions. Mol Cell Biol. *23(1)*: 216-228, 2003.

[108] Fujita N, Sato S and Tsuruo T: Phosphorylation of p27Kip1 at threonine 198 by p90 ribosomal protein S6 kinases promotes its binding to 14-3-3 and cytoplasmic localization. J Biol Chem. *278(49)*: 49254-49260, 2003.

[109] Sekimoto T, Fukumoto M and Yoneda Y: 14-3-3 suppresses the nuclear localization of threonine 157-phosphorylated p27(Kip1). EMBO J. *23(9)*: 1934-1942, 2004.

[110] Bunz F, Dutriaux A, Lengauer C, Waldman T, Zhou S, Brown JP, Sedivy JM, Kinzler KW and Vogelstein B: Requirement for p53 and p21 to sustain G2 arrest after DNA damage. Science. *282(5393)*: 1497-1501, 1998.

[111] Levine AJ: p53, the cellular gatekeeper for growth and division. Cell. *88(3)*: 323-331, 1997.

[112] Waning DL, Lehman JA, Batuello CN and Mayo LD: Controlling the Mdm2-Mdmx-p53 Circuit. Pharmaceuticals (Basel). *3(5)*: 1576-1593, 2010.

[113] Jin S and Levine AJ: The p53 functional circuit. J Cell Sci. *114(Pt 23)*: 4139-4140, 2001.

[114] Shieh SY, Ikeda M, Taya Y and Prives C: DNA damage-induced phosphorylation of p53 alleviates inhibition by MDM2. Cell. *91(3)*: 325-334, 1997.

[115] Assoian RK: Anchorage-dependent cell cycle progression. J Cell Biol. *136(1)*: 1-4, 1997.

[116] Huang S and Ingber DE: The structural and mechanical complexity of cell-growth control. Nat Cell Biol. *1(5)*: E131-138, 1999.

[117] Reshetnikova G, Barkan R, Popov B, Nikolsky N and Chang LS: Disruption of the actin cytoskeleton leads to inhibition of mitogen-induced cyclin E expression, Cdk2 phosphorylation, and nuclear accumulation of the retinoblastoma protein-related p107 protein. Exp Cell Res. *259(1)*: 35-53, 2000.

[118] Huang S and Ingber DE: A discrete cell cycle checkpoint in late G(1) that is cytoskeleton-dependent and MAP kinase (Erk)-independent. Exp Cell Res. *275(2)*: 255-264, 2002.

[119] Iwig M, Czeslick E, Muller A, Gruner M, Spindler M and Glaesser D: Growth regulation by cell shape alteration and organization of the cytoskeleton. Eur J Cell Biol. *67(2)*: 145-157, 1995.

[120] Bohmer RM, Scharf E and Assoian RK: Cytoskeletal integrity is required throughout the mitogen stimulation phase of the cell cycle and mediates the anchorage-dependent expression of cyclin D1. Mol Biol Cell. *7(1)*: 101-111, 1996.

[121] Gad A, Thullberg M, Dannenberg JH, te Riele H and Stromblad S: Retinoblastoma susceptibility gene product (pRb) and p107 functionally separate the requirements for serum and anchorage in the cell cycle G1-phase. J Biol Chem. *279(14)*: 13640-13644, 2004.

[122] Westermark B: Induction of a reversible G1 block in human glia-like cells by cytochalasin B. Exp Cell Res. *82(2)*: 341-350, 1973.

[123] Zhu X, Ohtsubo M, Bohmer RM, Roberts JM and Assoian RK: Adhesion-dependent cell cycle progression linked to the expression of cyclin D1, activation of cyclin E-

cdk2, and phosphorylation of the retinoblastoma protein. J Cell Biol. *133(2)*: 391-403, 1996.

[124] Huang S, Chen CS and Ingber DE: Control of cyclin D1, p27(Kip1), and cell cycle progression in human capillary endothelial cells by cell shape and cytoskeletal tension. Mol Biol Cell. *9(11)*: 3179-3193, 1998.

[125] Carstens CP, Kramer A and Fahl WE: Adhesion-dependent control of cyclin E/cdk2 activity and cell cycle progression in normal cells but not in Ha-ras transformed NRK cells. Exp Cell Res. *229(1)*: 86-92, 1996.

[126] Kang JS and Krauss RS: Ras induces anchorage-independent growth by subverting multiple adhesion-regulated cell cycle events. Mol Cell Biol. *16(7)*: 3370-3380, 1996.

[127] Schulze A, Zerfass-Thome K, Berges J, Middendorp S, Jansen-Durr P and Henglein B: Anchorage-dependent transcription of the cyclin A gene. Mol Cell Biol. *16(9)*: 4632-4638, 1996.

[128] Schulze A, Zerfass K, Spitkovsky D, Middendorp S, Berges J, Helin K, Jansen-Durr P and Henglein B: Cell cycle regulation of the cyclin A gene promoter is mediated by a variant E2F site. Proc Natl Acad Sci U S A. *92(24)*: 11264-11268, 1995.

[129] Barrett JF, Lewis BC, Hoang AT, Alvarez RJ, Jr. and Dang CV: Cyclin A links c-Myc to adhesion-independent cell proliferation. J Biol Chem. *270(27)*: 15923-15925, 1995.

[130] Kramer A, Carstens CP and Fahl WE: A novel CCAAT-binding protein necessary for adhesion-dependent cyclin A transcription at the G1/S boundary is sequestered by a retinoblastoma-like protein in G0. J Biol Chem. *271(12)*: 6579-6582, 1996.

[131] Fasshauer M, Iwig M and Glaesser D: Synthesis of proto-oncogene proteins and cyclins depends on intact microfilaments. Eur J Cell Biol. *77(3)*: 188-195, 1998.

[132] Roovers K, Klein EA, Castagnino P and Assoian RK: Nuclear translocation of LIM kinase mediates Rho-Rho kinase regulation of cyclin D1 expression. Dev Cell. *5(2)*: 273-284, 2003.

[133] Roovers K and Assoian RK: Effects of rho kinase and actin stress fibers on sustained extracellular signal-regulated kinase activity and activation of G(1) phase cyclin-dependent kinases. Mol Cell Biol. *23(12)*: 4283-4294, 2003.

[134] Lohez OD, Reynaud C, Borel F, Andreassen PR and Margolis RL: Arrest of mammalian fibroblasts in G1 in response to actin inhibition is dependent on retinoblastoma pocket proteins but not on p53. J Cell Biol. *161(1)*: 67-77, 2003.

[135] Hu W, Bellone CJ and Baldassare JJ: RhoA stimulates p27(Kip) degradation through its regulation of cyclin E/CDK2 activity. J Biol Chem. *274(6)*: 3396-3401, 1999.

[136] Metcalfe S, Weeds A, Okorokov AL, Milner J, Cockman M and Pope B: Wild-type p53 protein shows calcium-dependent binding to F-actin. Oncogene. *18(14)*: 2351-2355, 1999.

[137] Katsumoto T, Higaki K, Ohno K and Onodera K: Cell-cycle dependent biosynthesis and localization of p53 protein in untransformed human cells. Biol Cell. *84(3)*: 167-173, 1995.

[138] Takahashi K and Suzuki K: DNA synthesis-associated nuclear exclusion of p53 in normal human breast epithelial cells in culture. Oncogene. *9(1)*: 183-188, 1994.

[139] Bates S and Vousden KH: Mechanisms of p53-mediated apoptosis. Cell Mol Life Sci. *55(1)*: 28-37, 1999.

[140] Rubtsova SN, Kondratov RV, Kopnin PB, Chumakov PM, Kopnin BP and Vasiliev JM: Disruption of actin microfilaments by cytochalasin D leads to activation of p53. FEBS Lett. *430(3)*: 353-357, 1998.

[141] Kolber MA, Broschat KO and Landa-Gonzalez B: Cytochalasin B induces cellular DNA fragmentation. Faseb J. *4(12)*: 3021-3027, 1990.

[142] Lee YJ, Tsai CH, Hwang JJ, Chiu SJ, Sheu TJ and Keng PC: Involvement of a p53-independent and post-transcriptional up-regulation for p21WAF/CIP1 following destabilization of the actin cytoskeleton. Int J Oncol. *34(2)*: 581-589, 2009.

[143] Sakai N, Ohtsu M, Fujita H, Koike T and Kuzumaki N: Enhancement of G2 checkpoint function by gelsolin transfection in human cancer cells. Exp Cell Res. *251(1)*: 224-233, 1999.

[144] Wang WS, Chen PM, Hsiao HL, Ju SY and Su Y: Overexpression of the thymosin beta-4 gene is associated with malignant progression of SW480 colon cancer cells. Oncogene. *22(21)*: 3297-3306, 2003.

[145] Zou L, Ding Z and Roy P: Profilin-1 overexpression inhibits proliferation of MDA-MB-231 breast cancer cells partly through p27kip1 upregulation. J Cell Physiol. *223(3)*: 623-629, 2010.

[146] Hanahan D and Weinberg RA: The hallmarks of cancer. Cell. *100(1)*: 57-70, 2000.

[147] Sherr CJ: Cell cycle control and cancer. Harvey Lect. *96(*73-92, 2000.

[148] Jordan MA and Wilson L: Use of drugs to study role of microtubule assembly dynamics in living cells. Methods Enzymol. *298(*252-276, 1998.

[149] Lehmann KG, Popma JJ, Werner JA, Lansky AJ and Wilensky RL: Vascular remodeling and the local delivery of cytochalasin B after coronary angioplasty in humans. J Am Coll Cardiol. *35(3)*: 583-591, 2000.

[150] Lee YJ, Sheu TJ and Keng PC: Enhancement of radiosensitivity in H1299 cancer cells by actin-associated protein cofilin. Biochem Biophys Res Commun. *335(2)*: 286-291, 2005.

[151] Diez-Juan A and Andres V: Coordinate control of proliferation and migration by the p27Kip1/cyclin-dependent kinase/retinoblastoma pathway in vascular smooth muscle cells and fibroblasts. Circ Res. *92(4)*: 402-410, 2003.

[152] Assoian RK and Yung Y: A reciprocal relationship between Rb and Skp2: implications for restriction point control, signal transduction to the cell cycle and cancer. Cell Cycle. *7(1)*: 24-27, 2008.

[153] Hershko DD: Oncogenic properties and prognostic implications of the ubiquitin ligase Skp2 in cancer. Cancer. *112(7)*: 1415-1424, 2008.

[154] Signoretti S, Di Marcotullio L, Richardson A, Ramaswamy S, Isaac B, Rue M, Monti F, Loda M and Pagano M: Oncogenic role of the ubiquitin ligase subunit Skp2 in human breast cancer. J Clin Invest. *110(5)*: 633-641, 2002.

[155] Lin HK, Chen Z, Wang G, Nardella C, Lee SW, Chan CH, Yang WL, Wang J, Egia A, Nakayama KI, Cordon-Cardo C, Teruya-Feldstein J and Pandolfi PP: Skp2 targeting suppresses tumorigenesis by Arf-p53-independent cellular senescence. Nature. *464(7287)*: 374-379, 2010.

[156] Tanaka H, Yamashita T, Asada M, Mizutani S, Yoshikawa H and Tohyama M: Cytoplasmic p21(Cip1/WAF1) regulates neurite remodeling by inhibiting Rho-kinase activity. J Cell Biol. *158(2)*: 321-329, 2002.

[157] Yokoo T, Toyoshima H, Miura M, Wang Y, Iida KT, Suzuki H, Sone H, Shimano H, Gotoda T, Nishimori S, Tanaka K and Yamada N: p57Kip2 regulates actin dynamics by binding and translocating LIM-kinase 1 to the nucleus. J Biol Chem. *278(52)*: 52919-52923, 2003.

Viral Oncogenes and the Retinoblastoma Family

M. Geletu and L. Raptis*
Departments of Microbiology and Immunology and Pathology,
Queen's University, Kingston, Ontario
Canada

1. Introduction

The discovery of viruses is tightly linked to the most significant advances in Molecular cell biology, including cancer research. Cell division is a fundamental biological phenomenon, therefore it is not surprising that human cancer is an evolutionarily ancient disease, that attracted attention in early civilizations. The remains of a 4 million-old fossilized hominid show evidence of bone tumors (Diamandopoulos, 1996), while some of the oldest written accounts of cancer are recorded in the code of Hamourabi (1750 BCE), Egyptian papyri (1600 BCE) and others. Unfortunately, in ancient Egypt knowledge was the realm of priests, so the writings of the time attributed the etiology of disease to the "will of Gods". In ancient Greece, medicine was freed from the bonds of religion; Hippocrates (460-370 BCE) tried to use logical thinking to propose the humoral theory of cancer and his ideas influenced philosophers and scientists for the next ~1,800 years. During this time, knowledge of Mathematics and Physics was remarkably advanced; the acoustics of amphitheaters, built in the 5th century BC are as good as the best of today's structures. Still, these amazing minds believed in spontaneous generation of life, a theory that lasted till Louis Pasteur (1822-1895) who demonstrated that living things cannot be generated automatically (Javier and Butel, 2008).

In 1892 Ivanofsky and Beijerinck became the fathers of the new field of Virology by showing that an infectious pathogen of tobacco plants, the Tobacco Mosaic agent, retained infectivity after passage through filters of unglazed porcelaine, known to retain bacteria (Levine, 2001). These landmark discoveries were quickly followed by the discovery of the first cancer viruses, the chicken leukemia virus by Ellerman and Bang in 1908, and the Rous Sarcoma virus in 1911. Since that time, virus research and cancer research have been closely integrated, since complicated biological problems that constitute the basic mechanisms of life are highly conserved, since they cannot change radically once solved by evolution. As viruses need to use the molecular machinery of the host to replicate, they have provided us with valuable tools to study the host, including mechanisms of cellular replication, ie cancer. Historically, two classes of viruses, the retroviruses and DNA tumor viruses have been involved in landmark discoveries in cancer, and have played a fundamental role as models in molecular biology, as well as experimental cancer research.

* Corresponding Author

Early work by Sarah Stewart and Bernice Eddy demonstrated that the mouse polyoma virus produced in cell culture could cause tumors upon injection in newborn hamsters (Eddy et al., 1958). Soon thereafter, Vogt and Dulbecco developed tissue culture methods and it was shown that it could transform normal, cultured cells to acquire properties of cells derived from polyoma virus-induced tumors, such as growth to many layers, growth in the absence of anchorage to a solid support and tumorigenicity in syngeneic animals (Vogt and Dulbecco, 1960). At the same time, Simian Virus 40 (SV40) gained notoriety because it was found by Eddy to be a contaminant of poliomyelitis and adenovirus vaccines, which had been administered to millions of healthy individuals worldwide. The public health implications of this revelation provided the initial impetus for an in depth study of SV40 biology. Later work showed that SV40 DNA sequences as well as infectious virus are in fact found in human tumors and may have contributed to oncogenesis. The fact that SV40 uses mostly cellular machinery to carry out important steps in viral infection, made it into a powerful probe to examine many fundamental questions in eukaryotic molecular biology.

In addition to their importance in cell biology, due to their potent transforming ability, DNA tumor viruses have been studied extensively. In fact, work on the mechanism of neoplasia caused by these viruses has yielded a plethora of information on cell growth controls and led to the discovery of two families of antioncogenes, p53 and the retinoblastoma susceptibility (Rb) gene products.

2. Replication of DNA tumor viruses

The DNA tumor viruses belong in the papova (the name is derived from **pa**pilloma, **po**lyoma, Simian **va**cuolating viruses) or adenovirus families. They all have non-enveloped particles and both groups are highly tumorigenic in experimental animals.

Polyoma viruses cause disease in a variety of species, with a very limited host range. The prototype of this group is the mouse polyoma virus, but three polyomaviruses have also been described in humans: JCV, the etiologic agent of progressive, multifocal leucoencephalopathy, a fatal demyelinating disease, BKV, causing nephropathy in immunocompromised individuals, (Hirsch, 2005) and SV40, the contaminant of polio vaccines, whose prevalence in humans is not clear (Garcea and Imperiale, 2003).

The response of cultured cells to DNA tumor virus infection depends upon the species being infected. In the case of SV40, monkey cells support the production of infectious virus, which leads to their death (lytic cycle), whereas rodent cells produce only the early proteins, ie the proteins expressed before viral DNA replication has commenced in a lytic infection, and acquire a neoplastically transformed phenotype. Similarly, polyoma virus grows lytically in mouse cells but transforms rat or hamster cells in culture.

Viruses of the polyoma family have circular dsDNA genomes of approximately 5,000bp, contained in icosahedral capsids. Their genome contains two coding regions, the early genes, expressed before viral DNA replication in a lytic infection, and the late genes which are expressed after viral DNA replication is underway. Both transcription units are regulated by a common non-coding control region that contains the transcription start sites, binding sites for the transcription factors and the origin of DNA replication. The early region encodes the alternatively spliced transforming proteins large T (or Tumor)-antigen and small t-antigen, while the mouse polyoma virus also expresses a 56kDa middle tumor antigen, which is its main transforming protein. The late genes encode mostly structural coat proteins (VP1, VP2, VP3, Figure 1).

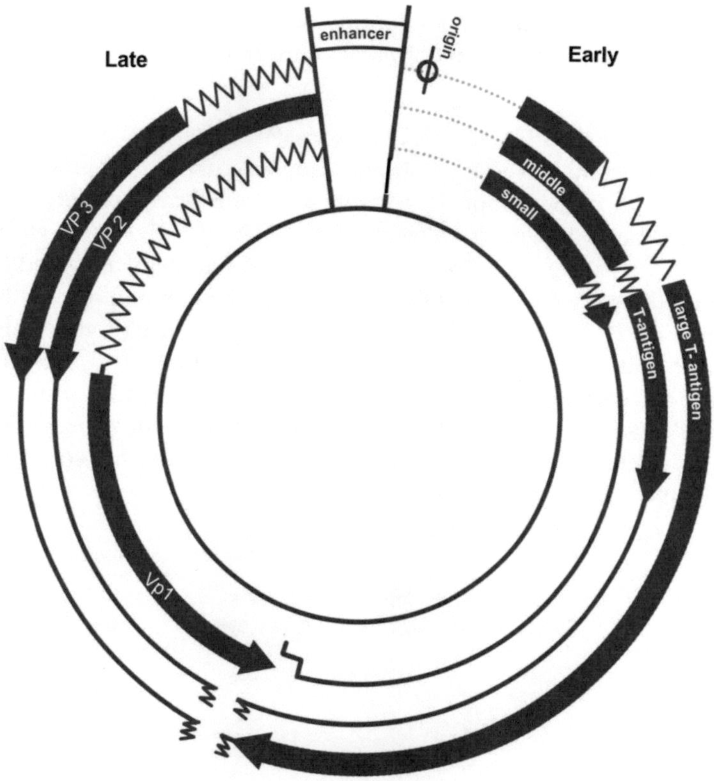

Fig. 1. Genomic organisation of the 5297 bp mouse polyoma virus. The early region is at the right and the late region at the left. The transcriptional enhancer and origin of DNA replication are also shown. Soon after infection, the differentially spliced, early genes (T antigens) are expressed (right side), followed by replication of viral DNA. After DNA replication, the late genes are expressed (left), coding mostly for the structural proteins, VP1, VP2, VP3. Squiggly lines indicate the introns (Cole, 1995).

In the host species, polyomaviruses spread by lytic infection of permissive cells. Lytic infection requires the large T-antigen, a ~100 kDa nuclear phosphoprotein which binds the origin and is essential for viral DNA replication [reviewed in (Cole, 1995)]. Polyomaviruses rely on cellular enzymes for the replication of their DNA, since their genome does not code for replication proteins. These proteins are confined to the S phase of the cell cycle, and the large T-antigens modulate cellular signaling pathways by interacting with a plethora of cellular proteins that promote cell cycle progression into S phase. Due to this property, the large T-antigens are also important players in the transformation of virus-infected cells. The most well-known interaction is the ability of the T-antigens to associate with, and interfere with the functions of the two tumor suppressor proteins, pRb and p53.

In non-permissive, cultured cells infection is abortive and neoplastic transformation of the cell may occur. Transformation requires expression of the early region, in particular the large T-antigen in the case of the human polyoma viruses (Fig. 1). The mouse polyoma middle-tumor antigen associates with and activates the cellular Src protein, but its large T antigen is also important in viral DNA replication, as well as transformation in certain systems. The tumor antigens are also key players in the highly efficient oncogenesis *in vivo* by these viruses, ie when virus is inocculated into animals or when the early region is introduced into transgenic mice.

Adenoviruses have linear dsDNA's of approximately 35,000bp enclosed in icosahedral particles with spikes on the vertices.The human adenoviruses infect and can grow lytically in human cells but can cause tumors in rodents and transform a variety of rodent cells in culture. Their genome is linear, double-stranded DNA of ~35,000 bp with a number of transcription units. Early after infection at least four promotors are activated (E1, E2, E3, E4), while at late times there is activation of the major late promotor, coding mostly for a number of coat proteins (Fig. 2). The adenovirus early region E1A and E1B genes are important in transformation of cultured cells and tumorigenicity, but E1A is also required in a lytic infection, for the transactivation of all other Adenoviral genes. E1A proteins bind the Rb family, while E1B associates with and inactivates p53. The adenoviruses display extensive RNA splicing, therefore it is not surprising that splicing was discovered for the first time in adenoviruses [(Broker, 1984), reviewed in (Shenk, 1995)].

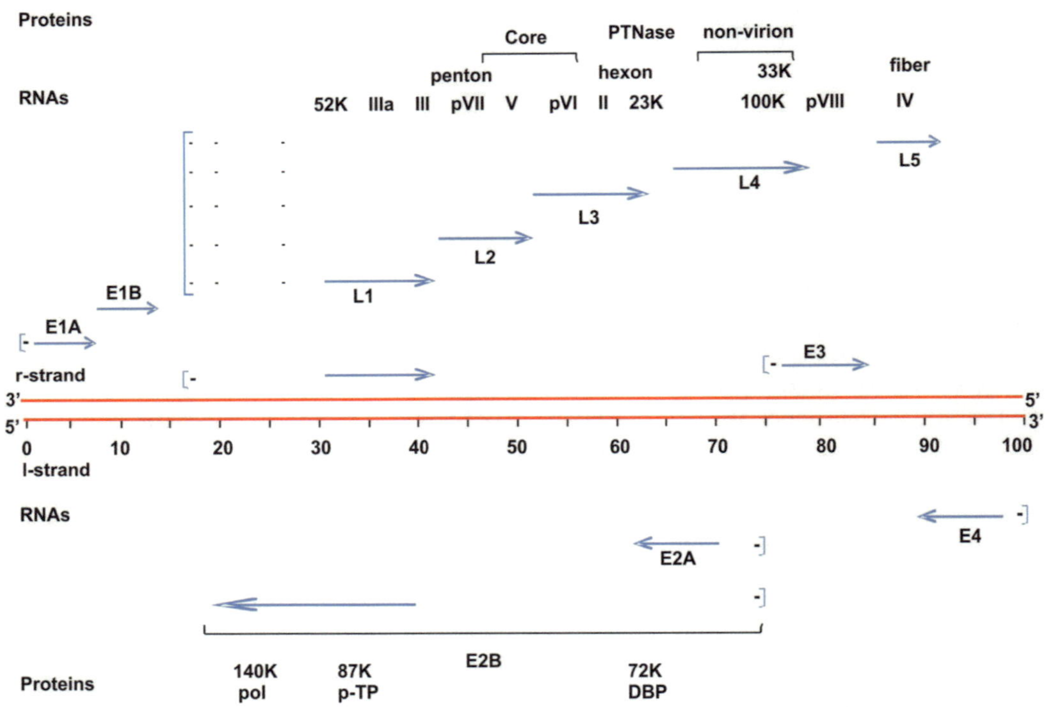

Fig. 2. Transcription and translation map of adenovirus type 2. The early mRNAs are designated E, late mRNAs are designated L. The main genes involved in transformation are the E1A and E1B at the left of the genome, giving rise to several proteins with differential splicing (not shown). (From Broker, 1984).

r-strand: rightwards transcribed, l-strand, leftwards transcribed.

The papillomaviruses comprise a group of nonenveloped DNA viruses that induce mostly benign lesions of the skin (warts) and mucous membranes (condylomas) in humans and animals. However, some members such as human papilloma viruses 16 and 18 have been implicated in the development of epithelial malignancies, especially cancer of the uterine cervix and other tumors of the urogenital tract. The papillomaviruses are small, nonenveloped, icosahedral DNA viruses that replicate in the nucleus of squamous epithelial cells. The virion has a single molecule of double-stranded, circular DNA of approximately 8,000 base pairs. The E6 and E7 are the main oncogenes of the high-risk HPVs. E7 binds with and inactivates Rb, while E6 binds p53 and leads to its degradation (Howley and Lowy, 2007)

3. Interaction of the DNA tumor virus oncogenes with the retinoblastoma family

The demonstration that DNA tumor viruses can cause tumors in animals led to an intensive investigation into the mechanism of tumor induction. The type of tumor that developed in an animal following viral inocculation often depended upon the site of injection; early findings demonstrated that injection of adenovirus-12 directly into the vitreous body of newborn rats, mice or baboons induced retinoblastoma-like tumors that expressed adenovirus gene products (Kobayashi and Mukai, 1973; Mukai et al., 1977; Mukai et al., 1980; Kobayashi et al., 1982). However, no adenovirus or JC polyoma virus was ever found in human retinoblastomas. Still, adenovirus research and the development of monoclonal antibodies against the tumor antigens of these viruses greatly facilitated the identification of cellular proteins specifically binding to the viral oncogenes. One of them was the *Rb* gene product, whose inactivation was independently demonstrated to lead to retinoblastoma formation in humans.

Seminal studies on retinoblastoma by Knudson *et al* (Knudson, Jr., 1971) laid the foundation for the tumor suppressor hypothesis. Statistical analysis of age and family history made him conclude that two independent mutation events are required for retinoblastoma development. It was later proposed that the two mutations occurred in the two alleles of the same gene, *Rb1* that is, retinoblastoma is a recessive cancer where one abnormal chromosome was inherited, while the corresponding, wild-type chromosomal segment was lost in the tumor cells (Godbout et al., 1983; Benedict et al., 1983). Genetic linkage studies demonstrated anomalies on chromosome 13q14, close to the esterase D locus (Sparkes et al., 1983). Cloning of the retinoblastoma cDNA followed and it was shown that it encodes a 110 kDa nuclear phosphoprotein (Lee et al., 1987). Additional studies showed that the *Rb1* gene from retinoblastoma tumors had deletions and mutations, consistent with a model where gene inactivation ie loss of function leads to tumor formation [reviewed in (Burkhart and Sage, 2008)].

Several groups tried to identify cellular proteins that bind to the E1A gene products. Branton *et al* developed a series of anti-peptide antisera and identified several co-immunoprecipitated proteins, including a doublet of approximately 105 kDa (Yee and Branton, 1985). Most importantly, these proteins could be affinity-purified from uninfected cells using E1A expressed in bacteria. This observation indicated that the 105 kDa protein(s) was of cellular, rather than viral, origin. Moreover, their expression did not depend upon adenovirus infection, or expression of any viral proteins (Egan et al., 1988). It was further shown that residues 111-127 and 30-60 of E1A were required for binding to the 105 kDa protein (Egan et al., 1988). A breakthrough finding followed: A monoclonal antibody was raised using as an immunogen E1A that had been immunoprecipitated from E1A-expressing, 293 cells, therefore potentially containing cellular proteins bound to E1A. As it turned out, this antibody recognised the 105kDa, Rb protein. These data demonstrated that the Rb was, in fact, the 105 kDa, cellular protein associated with E1A. This observation offered the first demonstration of a physical association between an oncogene and an antioncogene (Whyte et al., 1988; Lee et al., 1987). Similar findings emerged on the SV40 system (DeCaprio et al., 1988). Most importantly, it was soon demonstrated that TAg mutants that were unable to transform, were unable to bind Rb (e.g. E107K). These mutants disrupted the sequence LxCxE, the site of Rb binding which is present in the large TAg's of both SV40 and polyoma, adenovirus E1A, the human papillomavirus E7 proteins, as well as the TAg's of several other human polyoma viruses (Munger et al., 1989; Dyson et al., 1989). Taken together, these findings demonstrated the cardinal importance of Rb binding in transformation by these oncogenes [reviewed in (DeCaprio, 2009)].

Examination of Rb's function demonstrated that Rb is unphosphorylated in quiescent (G0) cells, but its phosphorylation increases as cells progress in the cell cycle (Buchkovich et al., 1989). It was later found that it is the cyclin D/Cdk4, cyclin E/Cdk2, cyclin A/Cdk2 and cyclin B/cdc2 kinases, shown to be required for entry into the cell cycle, that phosphorylate, and thereby inactivate Rb (DeCaprio et al., 1992). It was also demonstrated that the SV40-TAg binds the under- or unphosphorylated form of Rb exclusively (Ludlow et al., 1990), which suggested that the G0 form of Rb served a growth-suppressive function, which was overcome by TAg. In addition, overexpression of Rb inhibits cell cycle progression from G1 to S (Goodrich et al., 1991). Finally, transgenic expression of SV40-TAg under control of luteinizing hormone-β induces retinoblastomas and TAg co-precipitated Rb in lysates from tumor cells, supporting the hypothesis that retinoblastoma can develop by the inactivation of Rb function by TAg (Windle et al., 1990).

Thus, the loss of the Rb growth suppressive function can be achieved by: 1. mutation (retinoblastomas), 2. phosphorylation (cell cycle), or 3. binding to viral oncogenes. It was later shown that two Rb-related proteins that also exhibit features of cell-cycle regulators, p107 and p130, can also bind the LxCxE sequence of E1A and TAg (Ewen et al., 1992; Dumont and Branton, 1992).

Several laboratories have mapped the Rb sequences required for binding the LxCxE sequence. In fact, the two thirds, C-terminal region of Rb can bind E1A and TAg, and it is referred to as the large-pocket, while the central part of Rb (379-792) constitutes the small pocket (Kaelin, Jr. et al., 1990; Hu et al., 1990) (Fig. 3). The central part of Rb was the site of mutations in retinoblastomas, and these forms also failed to bind E1A and TAg. This observation offers a strong correlation between loss of binding to the oncogene to loss of function (Kaelin, Jr. et al., 1990; Pietenpol et al., 1990). That is, the viral oncogenes were found to disrupt a normal function of Rb, that was necessary for tumor suppression.

Further studies on the mechanism of tumor suppression by Rb and transformation by these oncogenes led to the search for cellular proteins that could compete with TAg and E1A for Rb binding. One of these protein families is the E2F transcription factors. In fact, the hypophosphorylated form of Rb binds E2F and using Rb affinity columns it became clear

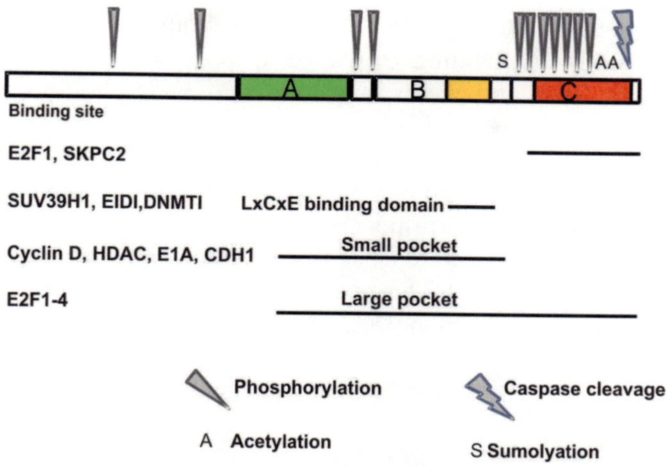

Fig. 3. A) The human pRb consists of 928 aminoacids. Deletion mutagenesis, as well as structural studies have uncovered regions that mediate its binding to individual partners. Most of them bind the pocket region. The Rb C-terminus binds specifically to E2F1 and this inhibits apoptosis. Rb can also be phosphorylated by CDK kinases as well as CHk2 (checkpoint homologue 2) and Raf 1 and this inhibits binding of most partners (Burkhart and Sage, 2008).

SKP2: S-phase kinase-associated protein-2; SUV39H1: methyltransferase, methylates lysine 9 of the amino terminus of histone H3; DNMT1: DNA methyltransferase-1; HDAC: histone deacetylase; CDH1: cadherin-1

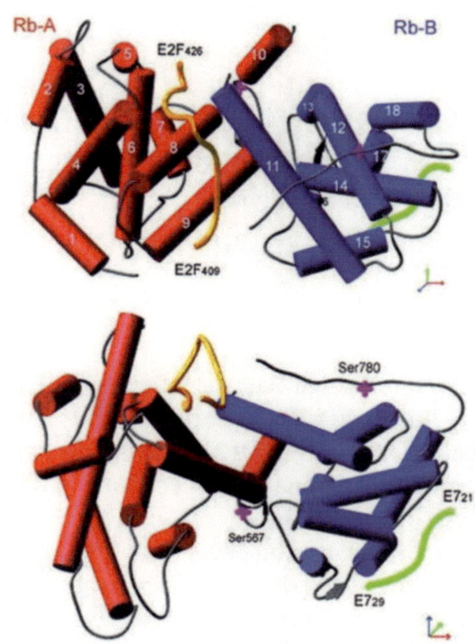

Fig. 3. B) Three-dimensional structure of the Rb/E2F complex. The helices of the A domain are shown in red and the B domain in blue. The main-chain trace of E2F is shown as a yellow worm (upper panel), while the main-chain trace of the papillomavirus E7 is shown as a green worm (lower panel) (Xiao et al., 2003).

that the viral oncogenes (E1A, TAg, E7) dissociate Rb from E2F (Chellappan et al., 1992; Chellappan et al., 1991). Rb binding correlated with repression of E2F transcriptional activity (Hiebert et al., 1992), and overexpression of E2F1 could promote entry into S phase in a manner similar to adenovirus E1A (Johnson et al., 1993). Therefore, the prevailing model is that E1A could serve to dissociate Rb from E2F, while the conserved LxCxE motif plays an important role in the high affinity binding of the viral oncoproteins to Rb. In fact, a minimal peptide of 9 residues corresponding to the LxCxE motif of HPV16-E7 could compete with Rb binding to E2F and to DNA (Jones et al., 1992). There is also evidence that TAg and E1A recruit the CBP/p300 histone acetyltransferase to remodel chromatin and actively start transcription (reviewed in (DeCaprio, 2009), Fig. 4).

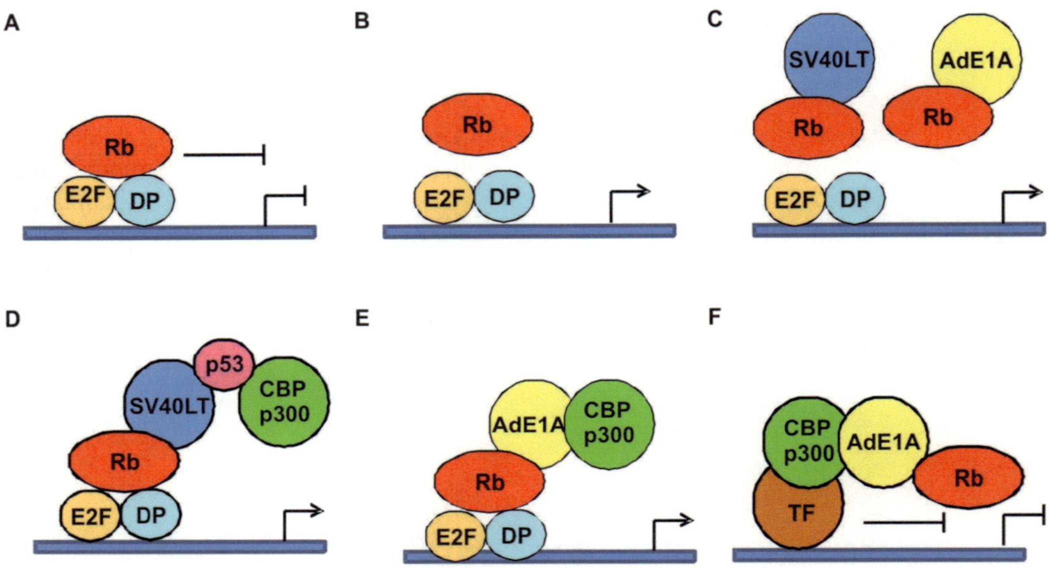

Fig. 4. Effect of TAg or adenovirus E1A upon Rb.

A. Active Rb binds the E2F/DP complex to repress transcription. **B**. Rb phosphorylation reduces binding to E2F/DP, permitting E2F activation. **C**. TAg or E1A binding removes Rb and permits E2F action. **D-E**: TAg or E1A can also bind the CBP/p300 histone acetyltransferase to increase gene expression. **F**. E1A can also bring Rb to CBP/p300 bound to transcription factors to repress promotors.

The crystal structure of Rb demonstrated that the A and B domains of the small pocket are bound to each other and are linked with a large area of highly conserved residues located in the fold between them. The LxCxE motif of HPV-E7 is bound to an exposed cleft within the B domain. The side chains of L,C and E make direct contact to Rb, which explains their high degree of conservation (Fig. 3B) (Xiao et al., 2003). Still, E1A and large TAg employ a different activity to displace E2F from Rb. The 100, N-terminal residues of LT form a J-domain, found in the family of DnaJ-Hsp40 molecular chaperones (Stubdal et al., 1997). The J domain recruits Hsc70 and activates its ATPase activity to promote chaperone activity. The J domain of large TAg cooperates with the LxCxE motif to dissociate Rb family members from E2F4 (Kim et al., 2001).

It was also found that E2F acts in a complex with another protein, the differentiation-regulated transcription factor-polypeptide 1 (DP1), which forms a heterotrimeric complex with E2F1 and cooperates with E2F for promotor binding (Simonson and Herman, 1993). Since the original cloning, a large number of E2F and DP molecules have been identified that play a variety of roles [reviewed in (van den Heuvel and Dyson, 2008)].

4. Other viral gene products interacting with the retinoblastoma family

In addition to the DNA tumor viruses, viruses from other families, both DNA and RNA are known to interact with Rb directly. Following are some examples:

The Hepatitis C virus is a positive-strand RNA virus, which causes persistent infections that can lead to hepatocellular carcinoma (HCC). The viral RNA-dependent, RNA polymerase NS5B forms a complex with Rb, targeting it for degradation and this increases E2F activity in E2F activity. NS5B contains a LxC/AxE motif which overlaps with the active site of the polymerase, and its interaction with and inactivation of Rb may be part of the mechanism whereby HCV infection leads to carcinoma (Munakata et al., 2005).

The Hepatitis B virus (HBV) also causes hepatitis and chronic infections that can lead to HCC. It codes for the non-structural, HBx protein which transcriptionally represses p21 and p27, and binds directly to cyclin E and cyclin A, leading to cell cycle progression (Dayaram and Marriott, 2008).

The Rubella virus (RV) causes developmental abnormalities and birth defects. RV is a positive-strand RNA virus encoding NSP90, a non-structural protein with replicase activity, which binds to Rb through an Rb binding motif (LPCAE). This association plays a positive role in the replication of the virus and it has been postulated that this contributes to RV's teratogenicity (Forng and Atreya, 1999).

The human cytomegalovirus (HCMV) belongs in the Herpes family and it can cause developmental abnormalities. HCMV codes for UL97, a protein kinase which can phosphorylate and inactivate Rb in a manner similar to the cyclin-dependent kinases. Moreover, UL97 is not inhibited by the CDK inhibitor p21 and lacks amino-acid residues conserved in cdk's that permit the attenuation of kinase activity. That is, UL97 is a functional ortholog of the cyclin-dependent kinases that is immune from the normal cdk control mechanisms (Hume et al., 2008).

The Human T-cell leukemia virus (HTLV) is the only human retrovirus shown to be the cause of a human cancer, adult T-cell leukemia. The Tax protein of HTLV (40kDa) is sufficient to transform cultured cells, and it achieves this at least in part through inhibition of a number of cyclin-dependent kinase inhibitors. Tax binds directly and inhibits p15 and p16, and it represses transcription of p18 and p19. In addition, Tax interacts with cdk4 and facilitates its binding to cyclin D2, leading to enhanced kinase activity, enhanced phosphorylation and proteasomal degradation of Rb, hence E2F activation. Tax also interacts with hypophosphorylated Rb directly, and this results in premature proteasomal degradation (Dayaram and Marriott, 2008).

A number of plant viruses were also shown to bind to and require Rb function for replication. Geminiviruses are small, single-stranded DNA viruses infecting a wide range of plants. The viral genome is encapsidated into two joined icosahedral capsids. The beet curly top virus (BSCTV) codes for the C4 protein which, upon transgenic expression in *Arabidopsis* plants can increase the levels of most cyclins and CDK's, CAK's and the proliferating cell nuclear antigen-1 (PCNA1). In addition, the Rb-related protein rbr1 and the CDK inhibitor ick1 are suppressed. Similarly, a protein of the Tomato golden mosaic virus, Rep, and the RepA protein of the Wheat dwarf virus are both able to bind the maize Rb-like proteins (Xie et al., 1995; Collin et al., 1996). Although the role of Rb in plants has not been firmly established, the fact that BSCTVcan induce cell division, points to the possibility that the effect of the C4 and Rep proteins upon Rb may be part of the mechanism of pathogenicity by these viruses (Park et al., 2010).

5. Consequences of E2F activation

Besides DNA tumor virus oncogenes, a large number of tyrosine kinases such as vSrc activate the E2F transcription factor indirectly, through activation of the CDK kinases. As a result, E2F is found to be hyperactive in many cancers. Transcriptional activation of E2F targets is achieved either through active transactivation or derepression of genes having E2F-binding sites on their promoters. A detailed Microarray analysis for E2F-activated genes yielded many targets, among which is a number of membrane receptor tyrosine kinases, such as PDGFRα, IGF1R, VEGF, and others (Young et al., 2003). In fact, it has long been demonstrated that transformed cells secrete autocrine factors, able to induce anchorage-independent growth to normal cells (Raptis, 1991; Ciardiello et al., 1990). These growth factors activate the membrane signalling apparatus, including the ras and phosphatidyl-inositol-3 kinase (PI3k) cascades, as well as the signal-transducer and activator of transcription-3 (Stat3) pathway. Following ligand binding, Stat3 binds to receptors of growth factors or cytokines and is phosphorylated on tyrosine-705 by the receptor itself or by the associated Jak or Src kinases. Two Stat3 molecules subsequently dimerize through reciprocal phosphotyrosine-SH2 domain interactions, the dimer migrates to the nucleus and initiates transcription of a number of genes (Yu et al., 2009; Raptis et al., 2009). Both the PI3 kinase and Stat3 constitute potent survival signals.

As a result of E2F activation, the SV40-TAg and adenovirus E1A have both been shown to activate and require ras (Raptis et al., 1997) and Stat3 (Vultur et al., 2005) for neoplastic transformation, as well as for the block of adipocytic differentiation (Cao et al., 2007b; Cao et al., 2007a). However, it is particularly remarkable that at the same time E2F is a potent *apoptosis inducer*, hence the high demand of transformed cells for survival signals, normally offered by Stat3, activated by the growth factor receptors. Therefore, direct Stat3 inhibition induces apoptosis of E1A or Tag-transformed cells preferentially, due to their higher E2F activity levels which promotes programmed cell death through p53-dependent or independent mechanisms. These findings underscore the importance of Stat3 the survival of tumor cells, and could have significant therapeutic implications (Fig. 5).

6. The Rb pathway in breast cancer

Although inherited, germline mutations in the Rb gene were identified mostly in retinoblastomas, Rb somatic mutations, mimicking Rb inactivation by the DNA tumor viruses have also been noted in a number of cancers, including breast cancer, so that, despite the fact that no DNA tumor viruses have ever been found in breast cancer, E2F is frequently activated.

Unlike the majority of cancers, the prognosis and treatment of breast cancer is significantly informed by a number of biomarkers, and the Rb pathway plays a prominent role [reviewed

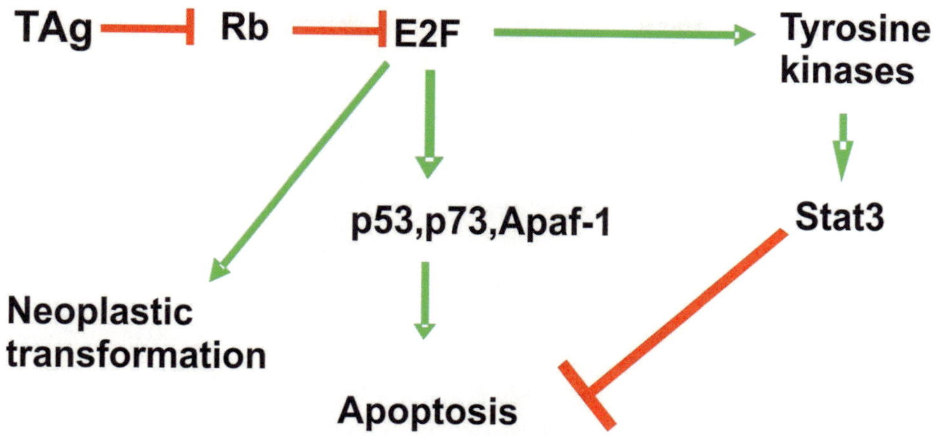

Fig. 5. E2F, activated through Rb inactivation by viral oncogenes, is known to be a potent activator of genes leading to cell division and neoplasia. Paradoxically however, E2F also induces apoptosis (through both p53-dependent and -independent mechanisms), but apoptosis inhibition would allow cell division to occur. In fact, E2F also activates a number of kinases such as IGF1-R and Src, which activate Stat3, a potent apoptosis inhibitor. As a result, Stat3 inhibition in cells with high E2F levels results in apoptosis (Sears and Nevins, 2002).

in (Musgrove and Sutherland, 2009)]. In particular, the status of the Estrogen receptor-α (ER) is an important determinant in treatment: ER-positive breast cancer has a more favorable prognosis and can be treated with selective ER antagonists (e.g. Tamoxifen) or aromatase inhibitors (e.g. Anastrozole), while ER-negative breast cancer is generally more aggressive, and with fewer treatment options. Still, a significant number of ER-positive cancers fail hormonal therapy and a great deal of effort has been expended in identifying pathways leading to Tamoxifen or aromatase inhibitor resistance.

In ER-positive breast cancer treatment, ER antagonists are effective at stopping cell division, indicating that such tumors are dependent upon estrogen for proliferation and survival (Musgrove and Sutherland, 2009). It was further shown that estrogen inhibition results in cell cycle arrest in the G0/ G1 phase of the cell cycle through attenuation of CDK/cyclin complexes at multiple levels (Foster et al., 2001). In particular, cyclin D1 is a direct transcriptional target of ER signalling (Eeckhoute et al., 2006). On the other hand, functional analyses have suggested that a multitude of cascades can contribute to acquired resistance to endocrine therapy, such as aberant ErbB2, Grb10 or Akt signalling (Miller et al., 2009), while p27kip1 and Rb inactivation can compromise the efficacy of ER inhibition (Cariou et al., 2000; Bosco et al., 2007). Specifically, a gene expression signature of Rb-dysfunction is associated with luminal B breast cancer, which exhibits a relatively poor response to endocrine therapy. Most importantly, recent reports demonstrated that a selective CDK4/6 inhibitor, PD-0332991 suppressed cell proliferation of a number of tamoxifen-resistant, cultured breast cancer cell lines. While ER antagonists in sensitive lines induce cell cycle arrest, CDK4/6 inhibition in tamoxifen-resistant lines induced a state having certain molecular characteristics of senescence in hormone therapy resistant cell populations. Therefore, PD-0332991 is an effective cell cycle inhibitor that could be especially valuable in ER+ breast cancers that are resistant to endocrine therapy, and is now being tested in phase II clinical trials (Thangavel et al., 2011).

7. Conclusions

Results on the mechanism of transformation by DNA tumor viruses have given valuable insights on the role of the Rb family in cell division. Evidence is now emerging that these conclusions are applicable to human cancers such as cancer of the breast, hence the Rb pathway may offer important targets for chemotherapy. It is reasonable to assume that the study of the viral oncogenes will offer additional insights into the role of Rb in cancer.

8. Acknowledgments

The financial support from the Canadian Institutes of Health Research (CIHR), the Canadian Breast Cancer Foundation (Ontario Chapter), the Natural Sciences and Engineering Research Council of Canada (NSERC), the Canadian Breast Cancer Research Alliance, the Ontario Centers of Excellence, the Breast Cancer Action Kingston and the Clare Nelson bequest fund through grants to LR is gratefully acknowledged. MG was supported by a postdoctoral fellowship from the US Army Breast Cancer Program (#BC087586), the Ministry of Research and Innovation of the Province of Ontario and the Advisory Research Committee of Queen's University.

9. References

Benedict, W.F., Murphree, A.L., Banerjee, A., Spina, C.A., Sparkes, M.C., and Sparkes, R.S. (1983). Patient with 13 chromosome deletion: evidence that the retinoblastoma gene is a recessive cancer gene. Science *219*, 973-975.

Bosco, E.E., Wang, Y., Xu, H., Zilfou, J.T., Knudsen, K.E., Aronow, B.J., Lowe, S.W., and Knudsen, E.S. (2007). The retinoblastoma tumor suppressor modifies the therapeutic response of breast cancer. J. Clin. Invest *117*, 218-228.

Broker, T.R. (1984). Processing of RNA. In Animal virus RNA processing, D.Apirion, ed. CRC Press), pp. 181-212.

Buchkovich, K., Duffy, L.A., and Harlow, E. (1989). The retinoblastoma protein is phosphorylated during specific phases of the cell cycle. Cell *58*, 1097-1105.

Burkhart, D.L. and Sage, J. (2008). Cellular mechanisms of tumour suppression by the retinoblastoma gene. Nat. Rev. Cancer *8*, 671-682.

Cao, J., Arulanandam, R., Vultur, A., Anagnostopoulou, A., and Raptis, L. (2007a). Adenovirus E1A requires c-Ras for full neoplastic transformation or suppression of differentiation of murine preadipocytes. Molecular Carcinogenesis *46*, 284-302.

Cao, J., Arulanandam, R., Vultur, A., Anagnostopoulou, A., and Raptis, L. (2007b). Differential effects of c-Ras upon transformation, adipocytic differentiation and apoptosis mediated by the Simian Virus 40 Large Tumor Antigen. Biochemistry and Cell Biology *85*, 32-48.

Cariou, S., Donovan, J.C., Flanagan, W.M., Milic, A., Bhattacharya, N., and Slingerland, J.M. (2000). Down-regulation of p21WAF1/CIP1 or p27Kip1 abrogates antiestrogen-mediated cell cycle arrest in human breast cancer cells. Proc. Natl. Acad. Sci. U. S. A *97*, 9042-9046.

Chellappan, S., Kraus, V.B., Kroger, B., Munger, K., Howley, P.M., Phelps, W.C., and Nevins, J.R. (1992). Adenovirus E1A, simian virus 40 tumor antigen, and human papillomavirus E7 protein share the capacity to disrupt the interaction between transcription factor E2F and the retinoblastoma gene product. Proc. Nat. Acad. Sci. USA *89*, 4549-4553.

Chellappan, S.P., Hiebert, S., Mudryj, M., Horowitz, J.M., and Nevins, J.R. (1991). The E2F transcription factor is a cellular target for the RB protein. Cell *65*, 1053-1061.

Ciardiello, F., Valverius, E.M., Colucci-D'Amato, G.L., Kim, N., Bassin, R.H., and Salomon, D.S. (1990). Differential growth factor expression in transformed mouse NIH-3T3 cells. J. Cell Biochem. *42*, 45-57.

Cole, C.N. (1995). Polyomavirinae: The viruses and their replication. In Virology, B.N.Fields, D.M.Knipe, and Hawley P.M., eds., pp. 917-946.

Collin, S., Fernandez-Lobato, M., Gooding, P.S., Mullineaux, P.M., and Fenoll, C. (1996). The two nonstructural proteins from wheat dwarf virus involved in viral gene expression and replication are retinoblastoma-binding proteins. Virology *219*, 324-329.

Dayaram, T. and Marriott, S.J. (2008). Effect of transforming viruses on molecular mechanisms associated with cancer. J. Cell Physiol *216*, 309-314.

DeCaprio, J.A. (2009). How the Rb tumor suppressor structure and function was revealed by the study of Adenovirus and SV40. Virology *384*, 274-284.

DeCaprio, J.A., Furukawa, Y., Ajchenbaum, F., Griffin, J.D., and Livingston, D.M. (1992). The retinoblastoma-susceptibility gene product becomes phosphorylated in multiple stages during cell cycle entry and progression. Proc. Natl. Acad. Sci. U. S. A *89*, 1795-1798.

DeCaprio, J.A., Ludlow, J.W., Figge, J., Shew, J.Y., Huang, C.M., Lee, W.H., Marsilio, E., Paucha, E., and Livingston, D.M. (1988). SV40 large tumor antigen forms a specific complex with the product of the retinoblastoma susceptibility gene. Cell *54*, 275-283.

Diamandopoulos, G.T. (1996). Cancer: an historical perspective. Anticancer Res. *16*, 1595-1602.

Dumont, D.J. and Branton, P.E. (1992). Phosphorylation of adenovirus E1A proteins by the p34cdc2 protein kinase. Virology *189*, 111-120.

Dyson, N., Duffy, L.A., and Harlow, E. (1989). In vitro assays to detect the interaction of DNA tumor virus transforming proteins with the retinoblastoma protein. Cancer cells *7*, 235-240.

Eddy, B.E., Stewart, S.E., Young, R., and Mider, G.B. (1958). Neoplasms in hamsters induced by mouse tumor agent passed in tissue culture. J. Natl. Cancer Inst. *20*, 747-761.

Eeckhoute, J., Carroll, J.S., Geistlinger, T.R., Torres-Arzayus, M.I., and Brown, M. (2006). A cell-type-specific transcriptional network required for estrogen regulation of cyclin D1 and cell cycle progression in breast cancer. Genes Dev. *20*, 2513-2526.

Egan, C., Jelsma, T.N., Howe, J.A., Bayley, S.T., Ferguson, B., and Branton, P.E. (1988). Mapping of cellular protein binding sites on the products of early region E1A of human Adenovirus type 5. Mol. Cell. Biol. *8*, 3955-3959.

Ewen, M.E., Faha, B., Harlow, E., and Livingston, D.M. (1992). Interaction of p107 with cyclin A independent of complex formation with viral oncoproteins. Science *255*, 85-87.

Forng, R.Y. and Atreya, C.D. (1999). Mutations in the retinoblastoma protein-binding LXCXE motif of rubella virus putative replicase affect virus replication. J. Gen. Virol. *80 (Pt 2)*, 327-332.

Foster, J.S., Henley, D.C., Bukovsky, A., Seth, P., and Wimalasena, J. (2001). Multifaceted regulation of cell cycle progression by estrogen: regulation of Cdk inhibitors and Cdc25A independent of cyclin D1-Cdk4 function. Mol. Cell Biol. *21*, 794-810.

Garcea, R.L. and Imperiale, M.J. (2003). Simian virus 40 infection of humans. J. Virol. *77*, 5039-5045.

Godbout, R., Dryja, T.P., Squire, J., Gallie, B.l., and Phillips, R.A. (1983). Somatic inactivation of genes on chromosome 13 is a common event in retinoblastoma. Nature *304*, 451-453.

Goodrich, D.W., Wang, N.P., Qian, Y.W., Lee, E.Y., and Lee, W.H. (1991). The retinoblastoma gene product regulates progression through the G1 phase of the cell cycle. Cell *67*, 293-302.

Hiebert, S.W., Chellappan, S.P., Horowitz, J.M., and Nevins, J.R. (1992). The interaction of RB with E2F coincides with an inhibition of the transcriptional activity of E2F. Genes Dev. *6*, 177-185.

Hirsch, H.H. (2005). BK virus: opportunity makes a pathogen. Clin. Infect. Dis. *41*, 354-360.

Howley, P.M. and Lowy, D.R. (2007). Papillomaviruses. In Virology, D.M.Knipe and P.M.Howley, eds.

Hu, Q.J., Dyson, N., and Harlow, E. (1990). The regions of the retinoblastoma protein needed for binding to adenovirus E1A or SV40 large T antigen are common sites for mutations. EMBO J. *9*, 1147-1155.

Hume, A.J., Finkel, J.S., Kamil, J.P., Coen, D.M., Culbertson, M.R., and Kalejta, R.F. (2008). Phosphorylation of retinoblastoma protein by viral protein with cyclin-dependent kinase function. Science *320*, 797-799.

Javier, R.T. and Butel, J.S. (2008). The history of tumor virology. Cancer Res. *68*, 7693-7706.

Johnson, D.G., Schwarz, J.K., Cress, W.D., and Nevins, J.R. (1993). Expression of transcription factor E2F1 induces quiescent cells to enter S phase. Nature *365*, 349-352.

Jones, R.E., Heimbrook, D.C., Huber, H.E., Wegrzyn, R.J., Rotberg, N.S., Stauffer, K.J., Lumma, P.K., Garsky, V.M., and Oliff, A. (1992). Specific N-methylations of HPV-16 E7 peptides alter binding to the retinoblastoma suppressor protein. J. Biol. Chem. *267*, 908-912.

Kaelin, W.G., Jr., Ewen, M.E., and Livingston, D.M. (1990). Definition of the minimal simian virus 40 large T antigen- and adenovirus E1A-binding domain in the retinoblastoma gene product. Mol. Cell. Biol. *10*, 3761-3769.

Kim, H.Y., Ahn, B.Y., and Cho, Y. (2001). Structural basis for the inactivation of retinoblastoma tumor suppressor by SV40 large T antigen. EMBO J. *20*, 295-304.

Knudson, A.G., Jr. (1971). Mutation and cancer: statistical study of retinoblastoma. Proc. Natl. Acad. Sci. U. S. A *68*, 820-823.

Kobayashi, M., Mukai, N., Solish, S.P., and Pomeroy, M.E. (1982). A highly predictable animal model of retinoblastoma. Acta Neuropathol. *57*, 203-208.

Kobayashi, S. and Mukai, N. (1973). Retinoblastoma-like tumors induced in rats by human adenovirus. Invest Ophthalmol. *12*, 853-856.

Lee, W.H., Shew, J.Y., Hong, F.D., Sery, T.W., Donoso, L.A., Young, L.J., Bookstein, R., and Lee, E.Y. (1987). The retinoblastoma susceptibility gene encodes a nuclear phosphoprotein associated with DNA binding activity. Nature *329*, 642-645.

Levine, A. J. The origins of Virology. Fields Virology 1, 3-18. 2001.

Ludlow, J.W., Shon, J., Pipas, J.M., Livingston, D.M., and DeCaprio, J.A. (1990). The retinoblastoma susceptibility gene product undergoes cell cycle-dependent dephosphorylation and binding to and release from SV40 large T. Cell *60*, 387-396.

Miller, T.W., Perez-Torres, M., Narasanna, A., Guix, M., Stal, O., Perez-Tenorio, G., Gonzalez-Angulo, A.M., Hennessy, B.T., Mills, G.B., Kennedy, J.P., Lindsley, C.W., and Arteaga, C.L. (2009). Loss of Phosphatase and Tensin homologue deleted on chromosome 10 engages ErbB3 and insulin-like growth factor-I receptor signaling to promote antiestrogen resistance in breast cancer. Cancer Res. *69*, 4192-4201.

Mukai, N., Kalter, S.S., Cummins, L.B., Matthews, V.A., Nishida, T., and Nakajima, T. (1980). Retinal tumor induced in the baboon by human adenovirus 12. Science *210*, 1023-1025.

Mukai, N., Nakajima, T., Freddo, T., Jacobson, M., and Dunn, M. (1977). Retinoblastoma-like neoplasm induced in C3H/BifB/Ki strain mice by human adenovirus serotype 12. Acta Neuropathol. *39*, 147-155.

Munakata, T., Nakamura, M., Liang, Y., Li, K., and Lemon, S.M. (2005). Down-regulation of the retinoblastoma tumor suppressor by the hepatitis C virus NS5B RNA-dependent RNA polymerase. Proc. Natl. Acad. Sci. U. S. A *102*, 18159-18164.

Munger, K., Werness, B.A., Dyson, N., Phelps, W.C., Harlow, E., and Howley, P.M. (1989). Complex formation of human papillomavirus E7 proteins with the retinoblastoma tumor suppressor gene product. EMBO J. *8*, 4099-4105.

Musgrove, E.A. and Sutherland, R.L. (2009). Biological determinants of endocrine resistance in breast cancer. Nat. Rev. Cancer *9*, 631-643.

Park, J., Hwang, H.S., Buckley, K.J., Park, J.B., Auh, C.K., Kim, D.G., Lee, S., and Davis, K.R. (2010). C4 protein of Beet severe curly top virus is a pathomorphogenetic factor in Arabidopsis. Plant Cell Rep. *29*, 1377-1389.

Pietenpol, J.A., Stein, R.W., Moran, E., Yaciuk, P., Schlegel, R., Lyons, R.M., Pittelkow, M.R., Munger, K., Howley, P.M., and Moses, H.L. (1990). TGF-Beta1 Inhibition of c-myc Transcription and Growth in Keratinocytes is Abrogated by Viral Transforming Proteins with pRB Binding Domains. Cell *61*, 777-785.

Raptis, L. (1991). Polyomavirus middle tumor antigen increases responsiveness to growth factors. J. Virol. *65*, 2691-2694.

Raptis, L., Arulanandam, R., Vultur, A., Geletu, M., Chevalier, S., and Feracci, H. (2009). Beyond structure, to survival: Stat3 activation by cadherin engagement. Biochemistry and Cell Biology *87*, 835-843.

Raptis, L., Brownell, H.L., Wood, K., Corbley, M., Wang, D., and Haliotis, T. (1997). Cellular ras gene activity is required for full neoplastic transformation by Simian Virus 40. Cell Growth Differ. *8*, 891-901.

Sears, R.C. and Nevins, J.R. (2002). Signaling networks that link cell proliferation and cell fate. J. Biol. Chem. *277*, 11617-11620.

Shenk, T. (1995). Adenoviridae: The Viruses and Their Replication. In Fundamental Virology, 3rd Edition, B.N.Fields, D.M.Knipe, and P.M.Howley, eds. (Philadelphia: Lippincott-Raven).

Simonson, M.S. and Herman, W.H. (1993). Protein kinase C and protein tyrosine kinase activity contribute to mitogenic signaling by endothelin-1. Cross-talk between G protein-coupled receptors and pp60c-src. J. Biol. Chem. *268*, 9347-9357.

Sparkes, R.S., Murphree, A.L., Lingua, R.W., Sparkes, M.C., Field, L.L., Funderburk, S.J., and Benedict, W.F. (1983). Gene for hereditary retinoblastoma assigned to human chromosome 13 by linkage to esterase D. Science *219*, 971-973.

Stubdal, H., Zalvide, J., Campbell, K.S., Schweitzer, R.C., Roberts, T.M., and DeCaprio, J.A. (1997). Inactivation of RB related proteins P130 and P107 mediated by the J domain of Simian Virus 40 Large Tumor antigen. Mol. Cell. Biol. *17*, 4979-4990.

Thangavel, C., Dean, J.L., Ertel, A., Knudsen, K.E., Aldaz, C.M., Witkiewicz, A.K., Clarke, R., and Knudsen, E.S. (2011). Therapeutically activating RB: reestablishing cell cycle control in endocrine therapy-resistant breast cancer. Endocr. Relat Cancer *18*, 333-345.

van den Heuvel, S. and Dyson, N.J. (2008). Conserved functions of the pRB and E2F families. Nat. Rev. Mol. Cell Biol. *9*, 713-724.

Vogt, M. and Dulbecco, R. (1960). Virus-cell interaction with a tumor-producing virus. Proc. Natl. Acad. Sci. U. S. A *46*, 365-370.

Vultur, A., Arulanandam, R., Turkson, J., Niu, G., Jove, R., and Raptis, L. (2005). Stat3 is required for full neoplastic transformation by the Simian Virus 40 Large Tumor antigen. Molecular Biology of the Cell *16*, 3832-3846.

Whyte, P., Buchkovich, K.J., Horowitz, J.M., Friend, S.H., Raybuck, M., Weinberg, R.A., and Harlow, E. (1988). Association between an oncogene and an anti-oncogene: the adenovirus E1A proteins bind to the retinoblastoma gene product. Nature *334*, 124-129.

Windle, J.J., Albert, D.M., O'Brien, J.M., Marcus, D.M., Disteche, C.M., Bernards, R., and Mellon, P.L. (1990). Retinoblastoma in transgenic mice. Nature *343*, 665-669.

Xiao, B., Spencer, J., Clements, A., Ali-Khan, N., Mittnacht, S., Broceno, C., Burghammer, M., Perrakis, A., Marmorstein, R., and Gamblin, S.J. (2003). Crystal structure of the retinoblastoma tumor suppressor protein bound to E2F and the molecular basis of its regulation. Proc. Natl. Acad. Sci. U. S. A *100*, 2363-2368.

Xie, Q., Suarez-Lopez, P., and Gutierrez, C. (1995). Identification and analysis of a retinoblastoma binding motif in the replication protein of a plant DNA virus: requirement for efficient viral DNA replication. EMBO J. *14*, 4073-4082.

Yee, S.P. and Branton, P.E. (1985). Detection of cellular proteins associated with human adenovirus type 5 early region 1A polypeptides. Virology *147*, 142-153.

Young, A.P., Nagarajan, R., and Longmore, G.D. (2003). Mechanisms of transcriptional regulation by Rb-E2F segregate by biological pathway. Oncogene *22*, 7209-7217.

Yu, H., Pardoll, D., and Jove, R. (2009). STATs in cancer inflammation and immunity: a leading role for STAT3. Nat. Rev. Cancer *9*, 798-809.